# HEPATITIS C

# FREE

## *ALTERNATIVE MEDICINE VS. THE DRUG INDUSTRY*

# THE PEOPLE SPEAK

LLOYD WRIGHT

PUBLISHED BY:
LLOYD WRIGHT
P.O. Box 6347
Malibu, CA 90264
(866) Hep C Free • (866) 437-2373
Lloyd@hepatitiscfree.com
www.hepatitiscfree.com

1st Printing March, 2002

## DISCLAIMER

The Reader or Purchaser of this book hereby acknowledges receiving notification in this Disclaimer that any opinions expressed herein are solely those of the company TRIUMPH OVER HEPATITIS C. None of the opinions expressed herein are to be relied on as statements of fact. Anyone having any questions regarding the success of the products described herein can contact TRIUMPH OVER HEPATITIS C at the phone numbers or email address noted above. Anyone who purchases either this book, or any of the vitamin supplements described herein, in reliance on either the book or the web site of TRIUMPH OVER HEPATITIS C, acknowledges that they are relying on their own investigation and not on any statements of opinion as to the success ratio of utilizing the treatments set forth in either the book or on the web site. The buyer of this book and/or purchaser of goods described herein acknowledges that they are making their own independent decision after discussing this matter with their current physician. No one should attempt to utilize any method of treatment set forth on either the web site of TRIUMPH OVER HEPATITIS C or in this book without first consulting their own personal physician for approval in utilizing the alternative health care methods discussed herein.

Cover Design by: Peri Poloni
HEPATITIS C FREE: ALTERNATIVE MEDICINE VS. THE DRUG INDUSTRY: THE PEOPLE SPEAK © Lloyd Wright 2002
ISBN 0-9676404-3-1
Produced and Printed in the United States of America

# *Dedication*

To every person who has had their life changed,
ripped apart, or ended by this silent killer, and
to all those who fight to open the world's eyes
to hepatitis C, the largest epidemic in history.

# CONTENTS

# *Acknowledgments*

It has been almost two and a half years since I published *Triumph Over Hepatitis C.* During that time, I have spent countless hours in phone conversations and have read through tens of thousands of emails. I have learned that what worked for me works for almost everyone who uses my program in a conscientious and persistent manner.

I am just a person who found the medical establishment to be disgusting and painfully ignorant concerning hepatitis C. I discovered that hepatitis C could indeed be cured without its sufferers having to go through the hell of taking interferon or pegylated interferon.

I want to thank everyone who wrote or called me to report his or her hepatitis C experiences. Some people traveled hundreds, even thousands, of miles just to see me, because they wanted to thank me in person for writing *Triumph Over Hepatitis C* and sharing my healing formula with the public. This is quite an honor. To all of you, I extend my highest thanks as well. I will always be praying for you.

I would like to thank my publicist Irwin Zucker for arranging speaking engagements and appearances on numerous radio programs where I could talk about my experience.

I extend my thanks to Donna Bible Larsen, who had the enormous task of plowing through reams of emails to dig out a good cross-section and arrange them in a coherent order.

Also, I give special thanks to my guest editor, Jessica Bryan, who proofread and formatted these very touching and enlightening letters into a comprehensive, understandable format. She is the light at the end of the tunnel in book production. Also special recognition needs to be given to Ryan Jordan, one of my staff for his exceptional understanding of the English language.

My staff deserves more praise than I can deliver. They answer the phone as much as humanly possible and work endless hours to help fight the Dragon!

And to my readers: This book is yours; you wrote it. Dragon, we are going to get you!

Lloyd Wright
February 2002
Malibu, California

# *Introduction*

Immediately following the terrorist attacks on the United States on September 11, 2001, an unprecedented number of people across our nation queued up outside the American Red Cross to donate blood to victims. These caring citizens were willing to stand in line for as long as five hours to donate blood as a way of showing their patriotism. But what we *didn't* hear about in the news afterward is the increase in hepatitis C virus that showed up in these blood donations. According to my research, of those people who donated blood nationwide during the immediate aftermath of the terrorist attacks, more than *double* the assumed ratio was discovered to have the hepatitis C virus. This is a dramatic increase. Judging by this recent finding, it would catapult the CDC estimate of 4 million Americans who have hepatitis C to 8 million.

My conclusion: Hepatitis C is on the rise in America. It is a rapid-growing epidemic, a hidden virus, and a silent killer. Many people are walking around with it who don't even suspect they have it.

Hepatitis C has a stigma attached to it, as do all illnesses that are not fully researched or understood. "Rumor has it" that people can only get this disease through intravenous drug usage (i.e. sharing needles) or promiscuous sexual contact. However, the truth is that most people get it at the doctor's office or the hospital through blood transfusions and surgeries.

In 1999, I published a definitive book called *Triumph Over Hepatitis C* that offers an alternative medicine solution. It is the most rewarding thing I have ever done. The book documents my battle with hepatitis C and how I overcame this insidious illness by creating my own

9

alternative health care regimen of herbs, diet and nutritional supplements.

The response to my book has been overwhelmingly favorable, so much so that my dedication to sharing this information with the public has kept me very busy. I have received many wonderful letters from clients that are inspiring and hopeful. People are hungry for knowledge about this "closeted" illness and how best to deal with it. These are people who have not been told the whole story by the reigning medical establishment, or who have been misled. They are people who have doctors who either don't know or perhaps don't care to find out more about hepatitis C.

For all its sophistication, conventional medicine is remarkably backward in its approach to healing. I want people to know that their doctors do not always have the answers. We have all been taught to place too much confidence in doctors and not enough in our own ability to heal ourselves. It is up to each individual to find out how to save his or her own life.

Many people have encouraged me to share these letters, in the hope that the myriad of hep C sufferers might find solace in the experiences of us kindred souls, as well as seek alternative cures that really do work! Out of the thousands of emails and phone calls that I have received, I have selected a variety for inclusion in this book. I trust they will serve to better inform and inspire the reader as to how this illness can be cured, and that life can be renewed for those who feel they have lost all desire to go on.

My first book, *Triumph Over Hepatitis C*, is considered by many to be THE bible on alternative medicine approaches to this illness. I have had people contact me who were so bad off they were considering going on permanent disability. Now, after trying my program, they are feeling so well they are not considering disability at all.

In this my second book, I will let my clients speak for themselves and tell you in their own words what my alternative health care solution did for them. I offer a wide variety of questions from intelligent people confronted with this terrible disease, and I have given my answers to the best of my ability based on my research. I have changed the names of the clients involved to protect the privacy of the innocent…or rather the healthy, as the case may be.

Here are just a few of the diverse comments you are about to discover in the following pages:

"I've got faith in your program and the innate healing powers of the body. We're not little statistical samples; we're the product of an incredible life force."

***

"Our so-called liver specialists know little about this silent killer."

***

"We are grateful to have found you on the Internet. Thank God I don't have to be made sicker to feel better by so-called modern medicine."

***

"A good day on Peg-Intron was a day I could get my head off of the pillow!"

***

"I actually cooked for myself this week, and I can drive again. I feel as though I have just gotten out of jail!"

***

"Everything happens for a reason. I'm so blessed to be a part of this patchwork blanket of recovery, and I am so looking forward to seeing others do the same."

***

"You, at least, have made yourself disease-free, and you have a similar distrust and disgust for what the medical profession passes off as treatment, which is really torture."

***

"The arrogance of the medical community is mind-numbing. How sad to say about people who take an oath."

***

"Conventional medicine is killing more people than AIDS, handguns, and traffic fatalities combined."

***

"Please tell me how bad I am. What does my biopsy mean? How high will the numbers get on blood work? Should I really be worried?"

***

"My brother got out of prison on time, and you'll never guess what the first order of business was. Girls? No! Seeing his family? NO! He came over here with a pad and pen to write down all the directions for your treatment. He read your book two times front to back, and left the book inside the prison for other friends who need enlightenment (as the medical staff insists inmates must take the interferon treatment or be written up disciplinary for disobeying an order. How lame is that?). My brother got written up and all he got was 30 extra days without commissary privileges, but after reading your book, he told medical staff 'no' and to just write him up."

***

This quote from a man in New Zealand, who flies to Southern California to purchase my products, is particularly inspiring: "There's something happening here. A month ago, I went to my gastro for a thorough checkup. He said he wouldn't have expected to see me in such good health. So, I'm walking on air at the moment."

***

Here is an email quote from yet another person who has wised up to the sad state of our American health care system: "We can let the medical staff know that indeed people can be cured by the natural way! Or do they really want people to be sick? In China, doctors are only paid if their patients are in good health. Isn't it wonderful to have doctors who really care about you and not always think about what they are going to earn?"

***

"Dear Lloyd, after talking with you on the phone last night, I got the courage to face this disease, grab it by the horns and beat it! I feel like there is finally hope. I thank you for putting your life story, words of encouragement, facts about our medical community's ignorance, and your love into words for others to share. I believe you have given so many a labor of love."

***

"After previewing your web site, I find that there may be a light in the far distance in this tunnel of despair."

***

"Don't let these MD a-holes get you down. They're protecting their zillion dollar 'good thing' at the expense of our lives. I work with a lot of them and on the whole (MOST, not all) they're mindless wonders with their self-esteem boosted up by years of overpay, graft from drug companies bribing them successfully to dispense their products, and the AMA boosting their 'credibility' and encouraging them to focus more on their own egos than on actual healing and curing."

***

Hepatitis C is a disease from which the body can cure itself, if given the right natural supplementation. Unfortunately, our medical system is designed to slice, dice and use synthetic chemical concoctions from the drug companies. The social anthropologists at the University of California at Berkeley invited me to speak on December 7, 2000, because they believe that the United States is in a backward, money-motivated medical malaise equal to the Dark Ages when it comes to the treatment of virus. Doctors are great if you have a bone jutting out of your body, but give them a chance to treat your virus, and they will take every cent you or your insurance company has, and you will still be sick.

If you or your loved ones have hepatitis C, I sincerely desire that you will find at least some of the answers to your questions here in this book.

Lloyd Wright

# ONE

# The "Silent Killer"

"Energy-robbing" and "liver-stomping" is how one of the clients quoted in this chapter best describes the quiet deadliness of hepatitis C, which is a very serious virus. It is a disease that causes much suffering and eventually death, if ignored. The severity of this illness is far greater than most people know. I talk to individuals every day who are in various stages of this tenacious virus.

Hepatitis C is called "The Silent Killer" for a deadly reason. It wears down the liver and other organs over many years, while its victims remain unaware of the damage the disease is doing, until one day they get diagnosed, either accidentally through a routine life insurance examination or after the disease has progressed to the point of making the person outwardly sick. By way of its insidious nature, Hepatitis C can cause a host of other problems in the body, including high blood pressure, diabetes, and thyroid, gall bladder, kidney and digestive ills.

This is not a sexually transmitted disease, a popular misconception. In reality, it is very difficult to transfer the illness to another person. But, unfortunately, a big stigma is attached to the illness in many people's minds, which results in unnecessary emotional suffering for those who have hepatitis C. The symptoms are bad enough without the attached stigma, which is born of medical ignorance.

Another misconception is that hepatitis C has no "cure," and you might as well give yourself up for dead. Of course, taking action as soon as possible is the best option for treatment to take the least amount of time. But it is never too late to begin treatment, no matter what the medical establishment tells you.

I offer to you the program that I researched, developed, and cured myself with after all the ignorant doctors and high-tech medical technology not only failed to help me, but also nearly killed me in the process. I do this because of my frustration with the medical establishment and the various governmental agencies that support it in keeping the people of this great country victimized by, and enslaved to, prevailing medical "wisdom."

Maintaining the myth that hepatitis C is a lifestyle issue keeps the populace from becoming inflamed over the limited attention and funding the disease receives for research. I offer to you what worked for me. No one should be sick or die from this virus. It is a disease your own body can fight, if properly armed.

The conventional treatment offered to us by the medical community is the man-made drug interferon and all its synthetic offspring. The success rate for this treatment is woefully poor, and most patients relapse in six to 12 months. The treatment itself is so horrific that if the side effects don't kill you, those around you will want to.

My program has a 97% success rate in reducing the AST and ALT to normal numbers for those who do even a portion of the program. For those who persevere through the entire program for the length of time needed, the viral loads come down to "non-detectable." The "side effect" of doing my program is that you will feel better in a very short period of time.

In this chapter, the reader can peruse a variety of letters and emails from people who, first, may have been surprised to learn they had the disease and, second, elated to discover an alternative program for treatment that works!

Lloyd Wright received all of the emails, letters, and phone calls recounted in this book from 2000 up to the present. They have been edited for clarity and content.

## You Have Changed My Life

Dear Lloyd,

This morning, at 6:30 a.m., I was driving to work, singing along with the Beatles. This may not seem like much to you, but before I started taking your products, I had altogether stopped listening to music at home and singing and dancing around the house like a fool. All because I'd lost interest, and because I had no energy. So as I was driving, I noticed that I felt energetic and happy, and in that moment I was very grateful to you. Just wanted to share it with you.

Just another little thing, right? You have changed my life.

Thanks,
Jane

## Finished Book the Day It Came!

Dear Lloyd,

From the moment I found your web site, I fully believed in you and your program. I ordered your book right away, and finished it the day it came. I was so excited to start the program. A little background about myself: I am a soon to be 41-year-old female, diagnosed in 1993 with hepatitis C. I could never figure out how I got it, honestly! I've never used drugs etc. I lived with this, seeing a liver doctor once or twice a year. He kept saying not to worry. My blood AST and ALT were high normal, and I had no symptoms.

Well, in December of 2000 I had an appointment with another doctor, because my original doctor retired. He matter-of-factly asked why I wasn't undergoing treatment [interferon]. I told him that no one had told me to. He was so rude to me! Said I needed a biopsy right away, which I did. My ALT was 65, my AST was 36, and my viral load was 2,000,000.

This was occurring right about the time I found your web site. I started really questioning how the hell I got this disease. Then, after reading about how a lot of people get it at the doctor's office, a light bulb went on. I remembered that in 1987 I received a gamma globulin shot because I was exposed to someone with hepatitis B. My two young children at the time also had the shot. They have tested negative for the hep C virus, thank God. I sweated that test more than anything. I was really pissed off to find that I received this virus from "the doctor's office."

Lloyd, you were so helpful on the phone every time I called with questions. I worked the program to every last detail, even the Natcell Thymus, which is very expensive. But I figured I'm worth it! I feel very fortunate that I could afford it.

Now the news we all are waiting for. I had blood work done last week, and after 3 months of your program, my ALT went down from 65 to 38, my AST stayed at 36 and my viral load went from 2,000,000 to 609,000! I was so psyched!

When I told my husband, he was so happy and my son, now 18, actually cried happy tears with me. My husband admitted to me that he thought the program was a hoax, but he's a believer now!

I can't thank you enough for all your hard work putting this program together. My family and I will always be grateful, as I'm sure many others are, too.

Looking forward to future blood tests and great results. I have to add this little piece. I am a very active, athletic woman. The past year or so I've felt tired and off kilter. Since starting the program, I have felt more energetic. Three weeks ago I tried out for, and made, a women's professional football team. My dreams of becoming a professional athlete have come true, with the help of you!

You're the best Lloyd,
Debbie B.


## Life Went from Horrible to Wonderful

Dear Lloyd,

If it wasn't for you, I don't know where I would be. I could not think straight, I could not drive; it was horrible. Now life is wonderful!

One month on your program and I drove 8 hours to Maine and I didn't even get tired. Then I went to Colorado and went skiing for the first time in years. I can't thank you enough.

After 60 days on your program, my viral load has dropped from 663,260 to 100,780. You are such an inspiration to me, and I pray for you every night.

Grace
(a 65-year-old female)


## What About Intimacy?

Hi there, I stumbled across your site while trying to find out what I can about hep C. My fiancé had an active encounter with the virus about 18 years ago and has remained primarily symptom-free ever since. We went to have blood work done to just make sure, and of course the test came back positive for hep C.

So, what do we do with this information? The R.N. at the health department strongly expressed her opinion that marriage/intimacy/children should not even be considered. I find this confusing because I have found other research that downplays the risk of passing the virus on. Is there anything you could offer in the way of advice?

Thanks for your time!<br>Lori & Tony

Dear Lori & Tony,

I have approximately 30,000. Most of them are married and have children. The only partners who both have the virus are ones that shared needles. However, I do have two couples that say they do not know how they got it.

All the research I have done indicates there is less than a 1% chance the newborn will contract HCV, if the doctor knows of the parent's condition prior to the baby's birth. I have a neighbor who has hep C, and she just had a baby a few months ago.

That nurse you mentioned needs her head educated. They call hep C "the silent killer" for a reason: Most people do not have symptoms for 15 to 20 years. By then, it has done severe damage in many cases.

I suggest doing the program outlined in my book. People who follow what I did have great results. It is definitely better than doing what your doctor is going to tell you to do.

I am here for any questions.

Lloyd

## Symptoms Almost Gone

I just found out that my brother has HCV too! It looks like I will be ordering more each month so that I can get him on the program. I got my most recent blood work back and it looks like I am almost cured! I have been feeling a lot better lately and my symptoms have almost gone away! I have actually been running 6 miles at a clip! My virus count is under 600, but I am still testing positive for HCV; I don't know why.

Lloyd, how many people do you know who are actually testing negative for HCV after going on your program? The reason I ask is not because I doubt you, it's because I don't see that many actual success stories on your web site. All I see are stories of how people are feeling so much better and their symptoms are way down like me. I know that you yourself no longer test positive, but how long do you think it will take for me to totally get rid of this hideous thing?

Donald

Dear Donald,

There are not that many reports of complete clearance on my message board for a number of reasons. I will attempt to explain some:

I get a myriad phone calls from folks telling me their story and updating me on their condition. Translating this information to the web site is a daunting task. Many people who have followed my program with diligence have stories of testing negative for hepatitis C. In the past, many testimonials came as emails that were easy to post to the web site. Phone calls are great because I get to talk with people, but typing them up for posting sometimes gets away from me.

I like to back up success stories with blood tests. Unfortunately, the doctors are often reluctant to give these test results to their patients. Please be aware these tests results are your personal property and if you request them, the doctors cannot deny you. If you send me before-and-after blood tests, I will post them for others to be encouraged. Be aware, the viral load tests and liver panel protocol has changed from ml. to IU. This makes comparing the past tests with current tests very difficult.

The bottom line is that most of us are just not conditioned to change our lifestyle and then practice the necessary changes for 18 months or the rest of our lives. We are brought up in a world where, when something goes wrong, we go to the doctor. We get a shot or a pill, and everything seems fine. Spending 18 months on a program whose costs are substantial is not something many people actually do. Sure, when starting, most are feeling very positive and dedicated to persevering with the 18-month program. However, as in many situations, the reality versus the ideal is often different.

Here are a few examples of the reality of the situation and people's good intentions:

One of my clients, one who will usually obtain a 3-month's supply of product, did not ask for more aloe when she reordered. When we spoke, she said she did not like it and hadn't consumed much of it. I spoke with her regarding the importance of properly prepared aloe, and she promised to try to drink some. This happens a lot with the tea as well.

Another person who had been on the program 10 months called and said his liver-panel numbers were in the normal range, down from over 200. He said that he felt good; in fact better than he had in some time, and believed he was well. Also, he expressed the need to relegate the money he'd been spending on the program to other areas of his life.

Often money is the major reason people do not see the program all the way through. They feel fine, the blood test numbers are greatly improved and their viral load is very low. A decision is made to save their money and go on about life as before, or hopefully with some new habits.

I also have several hundred people who only do part of the program, usually because of money, and most of these people feel better and their tests improve. There are many who experiment on their own and incorporate what they think is good. I am always open to new things, but I have found that people who do what I did have the best results. Time and time again I see this. I hear from people who start the program, then go off and do something else, then come back months or a year later and start over again.

Many people start the program and after a few months are feeling great, so they stop for a variety of reasons. They take a break for a month because of school, vacation, or other events in their lives that interfere with their commitment. I am in no way able to remember every reason I hear, but these are just a few. The part that disturbs me the most is that I see what happens to people when they do nothing. I do hope this at least in part answers your question.

Lloyd


Dear Lloyd,

Thanks for the lengthy response, Lloyd! That makes sense to me and I am going to make sure that I don't become another fallen statistic! Feel free to post this email correspondence.

Donald

## "Walking On Air" in New Zealand

Dear Lloyd,

There's something happening here. A month ago I went to my gastro for a thorough check-up. He said he wouldn't have expected to see me in such good health. My ALT seemed to have stabilized at about 90 after being in the 120-140 range for a long time. Two days ago ALT was 65! Never been that low since Noah was a boy! So, I'm walking on air at the moment.

FYI–I've been taking most of what you recommend but have been a bit slack about the dandelion and cat's claw teas. I've just started them again with a resolution to be more diligent.

That thymus and liver you sent all got thawed out last week when some clown unplugged my freezer. It would have thawed out over 3 days. Some thymus was still partially frozen so I'll keep taking it and see what happens.

I sure am enjoying the moment, though. Thanks for your part in it. I'll be in touch.

All the best,
Brett in New Zealand

## Your Book Was A Lifesaver

Lloyd,

I just wanted to thank you for the herbal supplements. Before I ordered them, my father was already doing "the herbal thing" with shakes and drinks and such. He recently went in for a checkup and got a "thumbs up" from the doctors. It's not that he's really doing "better," but they said it's certainly not getting any worse, which is good.

They said it's possible that he will live to be an old man. Wouldn't that be nice! I didn't think he would go out on his own and purchase your book, but I did know if I got it for him, he would feel obligated to read it. I'm glad I did. Without it, we may not have gone down the path we did!

Thank you again! Your book literally was a lifesaver!

Katherine

## Keep Those Statistics Coming In

Dear Lloyd,

I'm writing to let you know that we just placed another order and would like the discount if possible. Also, we wanted you to know that when we started Bill on this program on Feb. 12, 2001, his liver counts were: SGOT-141 and SGPT 366.

We had a liver profile done on April 25th and his counts were SGOT–47 and SGPT–25!

They were within the NORMAL range in less than 3 months! This is the first time in years that his liver count has been in the normal range. His hep C virus level is still greater than 850,000, but we are continuing with the program until it is zero!

Thanks so much. Yes, you certainly can put this on your message board. I want others to know that this really does work. I hope it will even encourage people to try this if they are not already on it or have doubts about it. We're looking forward to his next tests to see what the hep C virus count is!

Thanks,
C. D.

## I Feel GRREAT, Like Tony the Tiger!

Hey you!

Hope this finds you in good health and smiling. Me, I still surprise myself with more and more energy. This last weekend, Kenny and me built a 45 x 45 ft. turkey pen in the hot, hot sun, just drinking his Gatorade and me with my lemon water, and ya know I felt more hydrated than he did. I mean I feel "GRREAT!" As Tony the tiger says.

I have noticed that your herbs actually enhance my endurance. I mean it was 92 in the shade yesterday, and Sat. and Sun. we were in direct sunlight the whole day from 6:30 AM till 4:45 P.M.

Now that we've got the pen done, I can start raising my turkeys and have my year's supply of poultry (untouched by commercial breeders and their hormone additives). YAHOO! Just thought I'd let ya know how the herbs actually kinda kick in on their own when the body needs them to. You are soo grrreat, have a grrreat week.

Love,
Sue

## Peruvian Got Hep C After Brain Surgery

Dear Mr. Lloyd,

I'm from Peru, and I support my sister who contracted hepatitis C when she had brain surgery. That was last year, and she started with symptoms around June or July from last year. She is still in Peru. From what I know, she didn't have any treatment, and I don't want to lose her.

She needs to live with her kid who has Down's Syndrome. She started to feel not okay a couple of weeks ago. She is a little weak. We were trying to give her a good diet, but also we ignore many things. We can't afford to pay a lot right now, because it is me who is taking care of her financially. I need some orientation on how to help her, the way that she can overcome this. Please answer me to let you know whatever you need to give me a hand with this.

Sincerely,<br>
Roxana

Dear Roxana,

Your sister needs as a minimum the following:

Milk thistle 300, mg 3 times per day.

Lipoic acid 200, mg 3 times per day.

Selenium 400, mcg per day, no more.

Dandelion root tea, 1 quart per day.

This is a good start and it will help in a lot of ways.

In good health,<br>
Lloyd

## Impressed With Great Results

Dear Lloyd,

I hope this letter finds you well.

I just had some blood tests done lately, and I'm glad to report to you that my SGOT is within normal levels (23 R-F units or 11.04 U/L). Iron binding results are also normal (345 ug %). I went to a homeopathic doctor and she was impressed with the medications you recommended. She says they're helping me a lot. Thank you very much for your help. I think the big improvement is because of the medications you recommended.

Regards,<br>
Nathan R.

## Did I Mention I Feel Great!

Dear Lloyd,

I have been on your regimen of herbs, supplements, aloe vera and Natcell for a month and I feel GREAT. Prior to reading your book, the only option medical science offered a victim of HCV was interferon. I have read about that treatment and have friends injecting themselves 3 times a week with interferon. I don't <u>think</u> so!

It was a relief to find your book and discover that you felt the same, and that you also developed a natural remedy for this energy-robbing, liver-stomping disease. My symptom was fatigue. About 5 p.m. every day I would be exhausted. I have been following your program and diet of fresh foods, and the fatigue is over. In just 4 weeks, I feel revitalized. I feel GREAT.

I can only advise other HVC victims to buy your book and get on your program. It works, and in my case it worked immediately. Did I mention I feel GREAT!

THANK YOU,
Elizabeth

## Focus On Eradicating The Virus

Lloyd,

Thanks for the reply. Yes, my health is good and has been. I have high energy most of the time and am physically active as much as time allows what with family and work. My SGOT historically has been at around 49 and SGPT at 61. Within one month of using the dandelion tea my SGOT is in the normal range at 38. My SGPT has dropped to 54 after two months of using your cure and my

28

focus is on dropping it all the way to normal, as well as eradicating the virus completely from my body.

Mary

## A Subtle Message in the Numbers–A Story From Lloyd

"William" started my program in early November 2000, with these test scores:

Test Date 11/10/00–Collected 11/07/00
His ALT was 141
His AST was 79
His HCV RNA was 7,012,000 ml

In February 2001, he added the Natcell to his program, with the following results by March:

Test Date 03/16/01–Collected 03/13/01
ALT 117
AST 85
HCV RNA is 2,882,129 ml

In this case, we do not see the usual dramatic reduction in the ALT and AST associated with my program. We do however, see a dramatic reduction of the viral load, as is often seen with my clients. This reduction in viral load is equal to or better than what is seen with responders to interferon, without the hell associated with it.

Often, I am not aware of all of the habits of individuals, beneficial or non-beneficial. However, in this case I have been told that "William" stopped drinking six years ago, however, he still smokes cigarettes. He is currently reducing his smoking volume and plans to quit.

In the last six weeks, he reported to me that he was not feeling well for a short time. Often a cold or flu, virus, or infection can change the liver enzyme levels. Also, his doctor did not advise him to fast before the test.

When "William" started my program, he was contemplating disability due to his condition and is now not considering it at all.

These are very encouraging results and I look forward to sharing his next tests with you.

BLOOD TESTS ON FILE!

Lloyd

## Lowest Enzymes Since 1996

Dear Lloyd:

Thank you very much for your reply and information, as I have started on your treatment and I am very exited about it. I started your program in late January and went to the doctor yesterday for some blood work. My liver enzymes were lower than they've been since I was diagnosed with hep C in 1996. I hope with time and your treatment I can rid myself of this disease as you have.

Thank you so much.

Carl

## Impressed With Great Results–Phone Conversation

On December 20, 2000, I phoned a lady who has been on much of my program since August 20, 2000, to get the telephone number of a person she had referred to my program. During our conversation, she mentioned that in November she had blood tests performed. Her viral load had dropped from 650,500 to 325,377.

Her AST dropped from 50 to 30 and her ALT dropped from 35 to 30. This improvement took place in only 2 months!

I was prompted to ask why she had not called me to let me know of her results so I could share them with others. My client said that since she was the one who found my web site, bought my book, and obtained the products from me, then "she did it" and was not aware that she was required to report to me.

I only bring this up because people often quiz me as to why I do not have more results on my web site. This conversation is a real-world experience as to why I don't.

She gracefully suggested that if I want people to report to me, I should send them quarterly report forms. My solution was to write my book, *Triumph Over Hepatitis C*, make it available over the Internet, and establish a web site as a vehicle for informing people they can beat hepatitis C naturally.

It is imperative that I learn of my clients' success in order to spread the word. So please let me know what is going on, either through emails or by phone, and with your permission, I will post your comments and results.

Thank you!
Lloyd

## Now My Doctor Is Asking What I Take

To Lloyd,

Just a note for you, Lloyd, about how I am doing. Please post this on your web page for other people to read. I had blood work done last week and want to tell you that your program is great and working for me. I found out that I had hep C in June, and started taking everything you said, as nothing else was working. I had liver panels of:

| Date | AST | ALT |
|------|-----|-----|
| 07/16/2000 | 233 | 186 |
| 08/16/2000 | 122 | 186 |
| 10/16/2000 | 120 | 156 |
| 01/16/2001 | 94 | 124 |

I have been taking all of my herb teas, and the best, when I can afford it, is Natcell Liver Extract and Natcell Thymus. I know that this is the only way to go!

My doctor was always telling me to try his way and said this alternative program won't work. Now he is asking me what I am taking and wants to know more about it. Keep in mind; I just had hand surgery in the last two weeks, so if anything, my ALT and AST should have gone up. Thank you, Lloyd, for coming into my life. I feel Great!

Michael

## December 24, 2001
## Patchwork Quilt of Recovery

Many hellos to you, Lloyd and Aunika!

I have been way too elated to get this to you! I called you on December 22, my birthday, with the best news in my life; the results from my last blood test were in. The news was, and still is, the greatest feeling I have ever felt, my life has been changed forever. Just 5 months ago I thought all kinds of things all at once. I was so overcome by fear and confusion I almost gave up.

I've been a runner all of my life and this was not going to be any different, or so I thought. Something inside of me wanted to live more than I wanted to live. It was the spirit of God; only the spirit of God could have caused me to get results this fast, and my prayers answered, you go figure! After what the doctor offered me, I began a journey to find some help, some kind of sense of this whole hepatitis C thing.

I was scared to death; all I had was a doctor telling me that I had a bad disease. When I left his office, I never felt so alone. I sat in my car and cried very, very hard for a good 10 minutes; I'll never forget it.

About 2 weeks later, after reading all I wanted to read about the treatment plan offered to me by the medical people, I decided to get on the Internet. I found your web site and my husband and I ordered your book right away.

When it arrived at our house, I made a decision to follow every step you did took and by the grace of God, I feel better, look better, and have a better outlook on life than I ever did! And to all who read this, I'm not sitting down! Everything happens for a reason. I'm so blessed to be a part of this patchwork blanket of recovery and am so looking forward to seeing others do the same.

Thank you Lloyd, words are not enough. Your life helps others minute by minute!

God bless you and yours,

Kerry G.

## A More Reliable and Fun Sex Life
## Three emails from Shannon B.

Dear Lloyd,

I am newly engaged to an incredible man named Ben, who was told by his first doctor that he was in beginning cirrhosis stage and not to do anything for one year (that was

33

2 years ago). Last week, a new doctor said that the tests results were actually Stage 4 and the only treatment option available is transplant!

Is that prognosis a reality, or have other Stage 4s been able to regain their health? We are awaiting arrival of your book. By the way, a nurse at the previous facility let it slip that my honey was considered as a "control" for a new study coming out. No consent papers were ever signed...the joys of being self-employed and on Medicaid.

Shannon B.

Dear Lloyd,

This is in follow-up to our conversation of over a week ago. Ben said that he would write a testimonial in 2 weeks after we return from our honeymoon. He is quite overwhelmed with the stuff remaining to complete, and won't add another thing to his plate.

First of all, I am a doctoral-level scientist (neuro-behavioral), and am driven by data as an assessment of the worthiness of an intervention. Since beginning the Natcell Thymus at Thanksgiving, there are times when Ben has been like a different (well) man.

He began with the first 5 vials, taking them 2 times per week (Thurs/Sun). He found that he did not feel much different on the day he took the thymus, but consistently, he is feeling more vitality (in every way, I can attest to that!) on the second day, and then feels like he is "running down" on the 3rd day.

After speaking with you, we made the decision for that he will take it 3 times per week. We will track his labs and send you raw data, as it is available. Last week Ben remarked that he felt as good as he did 3 years ago, before he realized he was sick. He has to be careful not to overdo

34

it on the days that he feels normal again, and we'll let you know how the 3 times per week is working...thanks for all your help. You are an angel sent from God. Have a Merry Christmas.

Shannon B.

Dear Lloyd,

God bless you and Merry Christmas. Tomorrow we get married. We think the Natcell Thymus definitely gave us a more reliable and fun sex life!

Shannon B.

## A New Mirror Image

Hello, Lloyd,

I wanted to let you know that I received all of your products and began taking them. I passed by a mirror the other day and saw something that hasn't occurred naturally for so long that I was truly surprised. I had rosy cheeks, color in my face! It seems like I have been pale and wan forever! So this was a big deal to me. Also, for as long as I can remember, from 1 p.m. on daily, I have had incredible, mind-numbing mental exhaustion in varying degrees. This usually culminates in wondering if 5 p.m. is too early to get ready for bed and having to force myself to go through the motions of accomplishing much of anything, like cooking dinner, or bringing in a little firewood, or God forbid, going to an afternoon appointment. My day was pretty much over early in the afternoon.

So my point is that this did not happen. I didn't go to sleep until about 11:30 p.m., woke up at 4:30 a.m., stayed awake the whole next day without feeling the need to close my eyes even once, and didn't go to bed until midnight.

These are small things, but they're pretty important when they're gone. These little things are part of what constitutes quality of life. My "get up and go had got up and went." never to return, it seemed, until I started taking the products, (especially the live thymus.) So in spite of having the flu and a bad cold, I FEEL BETTER!

I am so looking forward to having blood work done in 3 months. Remember, my viral load was at 31 million, down from 66 mil, and liver enzymes all in normal range, just from taking the supplements from my Naturopath. So think what your program is going to do for me.

Thank you for your book, your web site, and for sharing what worked for you. Before I stumbled across your web site, I was getting all my supplements through my Naturopath (at her cost, no mark-up), as she is also my boyfriend's mother. The price I paid was the same as it is through the hepatitis C pharmacy, so anyone who says this web site was designed to sell product is just plain incorrect.

I appreciate having quality products all available from one source at really great prices. And that's all I have to say about that! I'll be in touch.

Take care,
Jane


## Subtle Changes for the Good

Lloyd,

Good morning. Hey, this morning my husband said something that really surprised me about the subtle changes he has seen in me, that I did not see or recognize. For the last 9 days we have had snow, tons of freezing rain, and temps down to 20 degrees by early A.M., and I have been putting on my winter clothes. Kenny said he noticed I don't

36

gag from the turtlenecks anymore, and he said I don't and haven't gagged in months when brushing my teeth either.

Ya know, when things go back to normal you kinda forget that, but he's right. Last year I fought shirts that were high around my throat, and brushing my teeth would sometimes make me gag (that intermittent nausea). Now here I have been dressing in the mornings and Ken said, "Wow, you can wear those again, huh?" I didn't know what he meant till he told me what subtle changes he's noticed with me (for the good). Cool, huh? Well, had to share that with you, since you are the king!

Have I told you "thank you" this morning? You stay well and strong.

Love, Sue

## I Thought I Was Going to Die

Dear Lloyd,

After 100 days on your program and a few other things, I'm jazzed to announce again a dramatic improvement:

| Date | AST | ALT |
|------|-----|-----|
| 7/14/00 | 88 | 158 (before) |
| 11/2/00 | 52 | 81 (after 100Days) |

And now I'm feeling much better. Following this regimen is automatic, day in and day out, knowing that I just may be able to lick this thing for good. My sleep still needs to improve, but after feeling like I've not slept for years before starting this program, getting a couple of good nights' sleep a week is a tremendous and miraculous improvement.

A few months ago I thought I was going to die. I am so pleased to have stumbled across your web site.

Toby

## Jazzed To Be Getting Better

Dear Lloyd,

I wanted to take a moment to give you an update on my condition. You were right when you said I would have bad days and good days.

For 20 years I really never felt right, and I never slept thoroughly. After being on the Natcell Thymus for almost two months, things have dramatically changed for the better. Now I have one or two days of feeling crummy and then I get a little REM sleep at night and the next day or two are just great, physically. Good, then bad, then good again. I just got your book back from on-loan to one fella, and it's going to someone else who has this dreadful virus. I also faxed info and your phone number to someone else to get the word out. I'm just jazzed to be getting better,

Tiger

## Headed In The Right Direction

Lloyd,

About two weeks ago, "Bud" had a blood test to check on how your program was working for him. His viral count was down to 740,000 from over a million when he was first diagnosed with hepatitis C. We found that news very encouraging. In the visit with the doctor, he pointed out that "Bud" was not cured, but that he is headed in the right direction. Thanks to your program and lots of prayers.

Kate

## Truly A Miracle

Dear Lloyd,

I just returned from yet another visit to the Lexington medical center, where a few weeks ago I had another viral count performed and guess what...I am clear of the virus! My doctor wants to do another count in three months to see if it is really true. He said if this was the same after three months, that it would be truly a miracle.

I believe that the herbs really helped. Thought I would pass that on to you.

Shaun

## What A Great Birthday Present

Hi you guys,

It's me Katie and it's my birthday! I just got my blood tests results and my viral load was only 28,000! In September it was 336,000.

I owe you guys everything and I love you all. I want you to know that I am going to tell the whole state of South Carolina about you.

God is good; you all are good. He led me to you. He has spoken through you, and now I owe my life to Him.

Thank you so much and Merry Christmas!

Katie

## Are Others Going Negative?

Dear Lloyd,

I ordered your book about 6 months ago. I read it within a few hours and found that many of the products you recommended I was already using. However, I was not using the frozen thymus.

My ALT has been normal since October 1999, but I was interested in taking it to the next level, i.e. reducing my viral load. This past September, my quantitative was 550,000. I have not used the frozen thymus due to my skepticism and inability to find studies to support its use.

I have read all the posted messages about others response. Please answer one question: are others really going negative on your program? I just want a straight answer or some evidence. I am strongly considering starting the full program in January 2001.

Thanks for your help and Merry Christmas,

Marty

Dear Marty,

People are going negative who do it long enough. That is a small number, because most people do not stay with the program long enough.

I have copies of many studies on the subject of thymus, and I can mail or fax them to you. Or, you can visit my web site at www.hepatitiscfree.com and click on "Why Thymus?" Call me if you'd like.

Lloyd

## Absolutely Devastated

Dear Lloyd,

I have just been told that I am HCV positive. I am absolutely devastated. At least I know why I have been so exhausted and where my aches and pains have been coming from. I have been feeling progressively worse for about a year now, and it was by sheer chance that they tested me for hep C. I feel really alone and scared. Your web site is really informative, and I am looking forward to reading your book.

Thank you,<br>Fiona

Dear Fiona,

You do what is in my book, and you will feel great. Your blood work will come back progressively better and, if you do it long enough, you will get well just like all the others who are persistent. You have nothing to worry about. That is the best thing I can tell you.

In good health,<br>Lloyd

Dear Lloyd,

It's so nice to hear from you. I told my mother about your book, and she can hear from my voice that I am feeling more encouraged since I found your web site.

I am so thankful to have found it! I get more blood results back in two weeks, and I don't know if I even want to know what the outcomes of the tests are. I think that I could quite easily become an ostrich right now and just stick my head in the sand!

I'll keep in touch—and thank you for giving me hope.

Fiona

Dear Fiona,

You cannot stick your head in the sand. You must simply do what is in my book and your life will improve. It could not get any better.

Lloyd

## Surprised by Quick Improvement

Dear Lloyd,

My husband started your alternative recommendations on 12/30/00. He doesn't see the doctor again until the end of February. We won't have scientific proof of anything until then, but I can tell you he looks and is feeling much better. His energy level has notably improved, and I'm surprised that happened so quickly. He has his color back. We are looking forward to a good report from the doctor in February.

Joy

## I Consider You One of My Angels

Hey, guy!

I cannot tell you how much I've enjoyed reading your book. I just received it 2 days ago and I cannot put it down. You crack me up. I laughed my butt off! I've been in a bad mood for 6 weeks. Your book is the only thing that has made me smile. I hate having this disease. Only found out 6 weeks ago, and I have been on a pity pot every since!

I went to the natural stores and picked up most of the items you mention. I am gonna follow every step you took. I had some dealings with the medical field myself. At the ripe old age of 23, I had a hysterectomy and still to this day do not know why. So I am staying as far away from them as possible!

Lloyd, again thank you for your support and knowledge. I consider you as one of my Angels! I'm very excited about your book. Thank you for doing the work for the rest of us! Friends in recovery,

Katie

## Healthcare System Different in Europe

Hi,

I started to read your book. There are so many interesting things. And it is a book from a patient to other patients. This is very important. I was shocked when I read that your health insurance cancelled your policy!

In Europe, we don't have the same system, and you can always go to the hospital, even when you are without a job.

Bye, Cinzia

## Going Through Crying-and-Scared Phase

Dear Lloyd,

Thank you for responding so quickly. I have another question. I was talking to a few doctors (some I know and a couple online), and I posed the question to them, "Have you ever heard of anyone cured of hep C?"

They all stated that they have never heard of anyone being cured of hep C. That scared me. I'm going through the crying and scared phase right now.

Well, thank you very much again, and I will look forward to receiving the information you are sending.

Sincerely,
Nikita

## Medicine Did Not Work

Dear Lloyd,

You're right when you say no one knows much about hep C. I have tried the medicine and, of course, it did not work. I have been using alternative medicine, but I'm having trouble finding the proper one for me.

I'm not sure what viral load means. Does it mean the higher the number, the worse you get? I'm not sure even doctors know the answer to this one.

I have so many questions. Anyway, thanks for listening. Looking forward to hearing from you again.

Suzie

## I Know There is More Out There

Hi,

I will get your book right away. I know for a fact that there is more out there than the medical community has to offer.

I had hep C 27 years ago and there was no treatment. A nurse gave me a book that suggested Vitamin B complex and a diet. I believe it saved my life, but I no longer remember much of it. Now the medical community uses some of these things.

Thanks again, Linda

## Hope to Recover My Father's Health

Dear Mr. Wright,

A couple of hours ago, the postman arrived with my copy of your book. Immediately I began to read it. As soon as I understand the recommendations and application to my father's case, I will order your products. I have a great expectation to recover my father's health.

Thank you,<br>Erick (in Mexico)

## Desperately Looking for an Answer

Hello Lloyd:

I am glad to hear that you are an over-comer and happy that you are interested in people who are so desperately looking for an answer. I am interested in your book.

I am a believer in the power of natural healing. This is really encouraging. Thank you for your time and help.

Janetta

## We Feel Great That Someone Cares

Dear Lloyd,

I just received your email. Thank you so much for answering so quickly! This news hit us hard because we have a two-year-old daughter.

After I got your email this morning, my whole body relaxed! I had not realized how tense I had been! You are a wonderful person for doing this! We feel great that someone cares.

I do plan on having my husband follow your program as soon as I read your book and figure out what to buy, how much he should take, etc. I hope you don't mind, but I may write again with questions. I am the question queen!

Thank you, thank you, and thank you!

Shaunti

## Improvement in Only Two Months

Lloyd,

My ALT has dropped significantly, from 212 to 69, and AST from 111 to 94. That's after only 2 months on your program. I didn't realize how sick I've been for the last 12-15 years until I started to feel better.

Thank you,
Eric

## We Are Scared. Please Help Us

Dear Lloyd,
Please help me help my husband. He has just been diagnosed with the virus. Please tell us where to start on your program. Should he start now? And what are the chances that he will fully recover. We are scared; please help us.

Joy

Dear Joy,
The best help I can suggest is to read my book and go from there. It will help you understand where you are and what you should do, and it works very well for everyone who does it. It is quite remarkable.

Lloyd

## Your Book Made the Best Sense

Aloha, Lloyd,
I found that I had HCV last July. I went in for chest pains. I had my biopsy last month and am still waiting to see a hepatologist. They said my viral count was 32.5 million and that I had genotype 1, stage 2, grade 2. What concerns me is that they also said that my left lobe of my liver was almost gone. Is this common? Could it be caused

by HCV? I have done a lot of reading, and so far your book has made the best sense.

Thanks, Doug

Dear Doug,

Your viral load is high, but that is not a problem. Stages are just an opinion a doctor makes by looking at tests, and I find that they vary and are not accurate.

It does concern me about the left lobe being almost gone. Did they give you a reason for that? It's hard to accept a stage 2 diagnosis with that problem. The liver is the best organ you have for regeneration. Much of it is done through adrenal receptors and your adrenal gland must be supported.

Lloyd

## The Light at End of the Tunnel

Dear Lloyd,

My husband has just been told he has hep C, and I have ordered your book. He is very sick with a cold and will not take any cold meds. However, I did go to the health food store and purchase some powdered vitamin C. He has been taking it for 2 days and still no relief. Is there anything he can take that will help?

Thank God for your web site. It is a light at the end of the tunnel. May God bless you and your family.

S.C.

Dear S.C.,

I have noticed that when someone has hep C and gets a cold or flu, it is usually much worse than if one did not have hep C. It will pass. The idea is to boost the immune system enough to overcome the hep C virus. It thrives just below the body's ability to fight it. A proper boost to the immune system usually works. That is why people on the program I outline in *Triumph Over Hepatitis C* get well. The cold will pass. Read my book. If you have any questions, feel free to call.

In good health,<br>Lloyd

## Got HCV From Blood Transfusion

Hello, Lloyd,

I read your book and am very excited, as I do not want to go for the interferon therapy. It just doesn't make sense to me to put poison in my system; Lord knows I have enough. I went to the blood bank to give blood for my upcoming back surgery and got the bad news. I had a blood transfusion in 1989, and I got the lethal dose.

I haven't had a biopsy yet and would rather not. My gastro says there is no rush, because it is such a slow-moving virus. But, I feel I need to do something, so I have been taking milk thistle, Thymu-plex and liquid liver caps. I stopped doing that, thinking what if I am doing more damage than good. I came to this conclusion when my gastro told me that there might be impurities in this stuff, as the producers are not under FDA regulations. He also told me that instead of buying this stuff, I should save my money and go out to a nice restaurant!

Anyway, after stopping, I didn't take anything for a while, and then I started taking dandelion caps. After a few days, my urine wasn't so dark. It looks normal. Is that good or bad? Thanks for your time,

Patty

Dear Patty,

Clean out the liver–clean out the blood. This needs to be done as a daily thing, as the immune system sends macrophage to the liver to kill the virus. It cannot get into the cell to kill it, so it kills the liver cell causing cirrhosis and toxins. Properly prepared aloe can be a very big help with this. Natcell Thymus feeds the immune system what it needs to kill the virus.

It is good that your urine is lighter in color. I suggest that you do as much of my program as possible. People who do, have the best results.

In good health,
Lloyd

## Tattoo Probably Caused Hep C

Hi,

Just recently diagnosed. Tattoo probable cause. For over 25 years, heavy drinking and marijuana usage. Although I have not yet had a biopsy, the elevated enzymes and other blood tests confirmed it. And because of the heavy drinking and marijuana usage, presumably I have a fair amount of cirrhosis. I have flu-like symptoms, low energy, constant mild fever, but no yellow skin. I'm 46 years of age, overweight, and my blood sugar is marginally type-2 onset diabetes.

You mentioned you have no trace of the hepatitis C virus. Your book also mentions that Dr. Stuart Larson claims that the Natcell Liver repairs the liver; it did not reduce the viral count.

Overall, I am very impressed with you and your crusade toward wellness. I am favorably considering your treatment regimen without the use of interferon.

Your thoughts and comments would be greatly appreciated.

Sincerely,
Tom

Dear Tom,

Dr. Stuart Larson was referring to the Natcell Liver, not the thymus. I have approximately 30,000 clients. All of them experience a drop in the viral load; 97% of them have a 50% to 90% drop in 2 to 4 months.

Viral hepatitis affects the pancreas in many people. Most of my clients with blood-sugar problems have their problems go away after a while on the thymus. But for some who are worse, I recommend the Natcell pancreas. It has actually reversed diabetes in all the people who have tried it. The problem occurs in the pancreas and live-cell therapy does an incredible repair job.

If, perhaps, you read my book again, you will be able to see when I took interferon, dates, amount, etc. No, I did not take it during the 18 months I was on my alternative program.

I did not do viral load tests during my treatment, as I had no insurance. I thought I made that clear. I had one at UCLA on April 10, 1997. I have had some since then, and I am still non-detected. I am feeling much better after the Natcell Thymus. I think Dr. Finnegan explained that in the foreword.

I did not mention exercise. *Triumph Over Hepatitis C* was my first book, and it is very hard to write a book and get everything in it. I went to work, which I can assure you is more than exercise. I sweated a lot; it is very important.

I stopped taking thymus after UCLA declared me non-detected. I still take it every once in a while, as much of it passes through here. It is like sex, hard to resist.

I suggest doing what you can; it helps. I hope that I answered every question. If not, I am here.

Lloyd

## After Transplant, Still Has Hep C

Dear Lloyd,

My husband just had a liver transplant about 9 months ago, but of course he still has hepatitis C. He is on many different medications, and I am wondering if your program or treatment works on people who have had a liver transplant due to hepatitis C. If you could, please reply to this letter. I will be very grateful that you have taken the time to help me give my husband a chance.

Thank you so very much,<br>Colleen

Dear Colleen,

I have been told that liver transplant recipients are on special immune-system suppressants.

Most of my program is an immune-system enhancing program. I have spoken with several people who have liver transplants, and many who have had two. I am not sure what the body process would be with my program and the new liver. Personally, I think it would be good, but I do not know, and I can guarantee you that no doctor knows.

If I were you, I would start him on a small amount of milk thistle and see what, if any, negative side effects occur. Then I would try some dandelion tea. I would try a small amount of selenium. I would try a little thymus. Of course, you should also ask his doctor to monitor him.

Please let me know what your doctor thinks and whether or not your husband is willing to try this, as it may work well on someone in his position. But again, I do not have any experience with this type of case. Wish you could have found me first, but we can go from here.

Lloyd

## Thanks From WFAN in New York

Dear Lloyd,

Thank you very much for doing the interview this past Sunday. As you heard, we have a responsive audience and we had many people call after the interview wanting your web site address. Hopefully, you will hear from some folks.

Bob Salter

## Does This TRULY Work?

Dear Lloyd,

I'm going to ask you an honest question, and I pray to God that you're telling me the truth because my husband's life is at stake. Does this truly work? And why aren't you telling the world about this on T.V.? Excuse my forwardness, but I need to be up-front. I have read your book, bought the milk thistle, and I pray to God that it works.

Please tell me the truth.<br>Mary

Dear Mary,

If you've already read my book, perhaps you should read it again. In the acknowledgements, I write that I have been on TV and radio. Just this month, I have been on 14 radio shows that were heard by millions. Two were broadcast around the world on satellites and the Internet.

Changing the way people think is a lot more difficult than you can imagine. I have been spending every waking hour on a crusade. I have the number one web site on AOL under hepatitis C. They are placed by popularity. I spend every cent I have spreading the word. Have you been sleeping? Have you read my message board?

Yes, it is TRUE!

Lloyd

## How About Hepatitis B?

Dear Lloyd,

Is this treatment effective on chronic Hep B also?

Chris

Dear Chris,

Yes, depending on how long you have had hep B and how much damage has been done. That will be the determining factor as to how long it will take. Most people with hep B have had complete recovery in a few months. A few who had it for many years and were in cirrhosis take longer.

My program can help and you will feel good while doing it.

Lloyd

## Hope to Rid Myself of This Disease

Dear Lloyd,

Thank you very much for your reply and information, as I have started on your treatment, and I am very excited about it. I started it in late January and when went to the doctor yesterday for some blood work, my liver enzymes were lower than they have been since I was diagnosed with hep C in 1996. I hope with time and your treatment I can rid myself of this disease, as you have. I will be chatting with you and hopefully getting herbs in the days and months to come. Thank you so much.

Cal

## Your Story Is Incredible and So Inspiring

Dear Lloyd.

I got your book recently and have been avidly reading it since. Your story is incredible and it is so inspiring that your goal is to help other sufferers to have a normal life again. I am mailing the book to my parents in Australia, and I will order another one for myself here in NYC. My Mum is most anxious to put my Dad on your regimen.

Sincerely,<br>Sheryl

## A Note of Thanks

Dear Lloyd,

As always, thanks for the work that you do and for taking the time to share your experiences and triumph over hep C. May God bless you and all those who contribute to your efforts.

George

## Met Some Wacky Medical Professionals

Dear Lloyd!

I received my first shipment of thymus yesterday. I have to say I felt like Goldie Hawn in *Death Becomes Her* when Isabella Rosellini hands her the magic bottle and says, "Live forever." Do you know that flick? Anyhow, nothing so dramatic happened, but I feel like I did something right, like it was something that's gonna help. It's the only thing that has really made sense to me after all the BS I've run into over the past year.

Tonight I see a new ND that has agreed on the phlebotomies (at last). I did ditch the homeopath last week. I'm sure he would have helped me down the road, but as you know this is a lonely road with a dead end if you don't try to help yourself as quickly as possible.

So wish me luck. I'm so glad to have hooked up with someone who truly understands this disease and cares about other people.

Did I tell you about the doctor I spoke to about thymus who said it could be linked to "mad cow disease"? I'm telling you, I've met some of the wackiest medical professionals out there.

As ever,
Vickie

Dear Vickie,

Check out the article on my message board from Russia. They have rediscovered live cell thymus. I like your description. I did not see that movie, but Goldie Hawn lives down the street from me and I usually enjoy her movies.

Feel better,
Lloyd

## Hep C Will Not Win This Battle, I Will

Dear Lloyd,

My name is Francine. I'm 33 years old and learned that I had the disease January 1998. Since then my life has been a living hell. My ALT and AST went bouncing from one level to another.

I was just surfing your web site, and when I read the messages from other people my eyes were in tears. It almost made me forget that I had the disease myself. And there I was, trying to find in the letters posted in the messages section which herb would come back the most in those stories to be able to help others.

Then I thought, it is so easy to want to find solutions for others instead of for ourselves. I have learned, and am still learning, to calm myself as much as possible when I'm under stress.

I talk to the disease and say, "You will not win this battle, I will." Positive thoughts are also very important. I would like to know the price of your book, since I read so many good comments on it.

Thanks for devoting your time and energy to trying to find the best solutions for infected people like us.

Take care,
Francine

# TWO

## GOING OUT ON A LIMB
## WHERE THE FRUIT IS

I like Mark Twain's philosophy: "Why not go out on a limb? That's where all the fruit is."

Our nation prides itself on its pioneer spirit, which the American writer and philosopher Mark Twain exemplifies. He rose to fame when America's pioneers were pushing farther and farther west, braving the unknown to create a better way of life. That's how I think of this chapter, as a brave new journey on an alternative healing path for hepatitis C sufferers. It is a path that with rugged perseverance can get you to your destination–freedom from hepatitis C.

This chapter contains those cries of joy that our early American pioneers must have felt. California's state motto is "eureka!" which our early settlers shouted when they migrated to the west coast. "Eureka" means "I have found it." As you can see from the quote at the beginning of this chapter, even some physicians are opening up to my alternative solution for triumph over hepatitis C. And as you will read from the many letters below, my clients are shouting "eureka" from the rooftop!

### Pakistani Doctor Seeks Herbal Cures

Dear Sir,

I have visited your web site and am interested to import the herbal remedies for HCV+ patients.

I am a homeopathic physician and am treating HCV+ patients from 1996. A lot of my patients have been cured. I want to add more herbal remedies with homeopathic treatment. I want to increase my cure rate, so I will purchase your products.

Best regards,
Dr. Muhammad Tenveer in Pakistan

## Another Doctor Branches Out

Dear Lloyd,

Your web site is excellent and works well for individuals looking for the kind of help you offer.

Our classmate Dr. Virender Soldi introduced Ayurvedic medicine at Bastyr, and it appeared to me that Indian herbal medicine was the leader in treating the liver. As I recall, Virender said that hepatitis could only be legally treated in India by herbs because it was much more effective than allopathic or homeopathic medical protocols.

I am recommending my present hepatitis patients to view your site.

Sincerely,
J. Mark Tillotson, N.D.

## The Results Are In

Hey, you all!

It has been six months since my last PCR test and I just got my new test results today! According to my gastroenterologist, I am no longer his patient! I am HCV NEGATIVE! I hope this gives you guys hope that it can be done.

He told me I could be re-infected if I partook in risky behavior, but that won't happen!

"Joey"

## Godzilla-Type Cure!

Dear Lloyd

I want to let you know I have a friend named Joel who had hep C. He went on Natcell and all the herbs and, basically, he told me he just went on a "Godzilla-type" remedy. He took Natcell, frozen thymus, and the frozen liver for about a month along with Transfactor. He went to his doctor and had extensive blood work done, and the doctor said he no longer has hep C.

They could not find a trace. Lloyd, this guy couldn't even get out of bed in the morning. He doesn't have a computer, so I am delivering the message. I am going to have my blood work done soon after the holidays and see how far I have come along. I know one thing is for sure, I do feel a whole lot better, and I am expecting to hear better news about my condition with hep C.

Thanx a million and God bless you, Lloyd.

Mark R.<br>Detroit, Michigan

Dear Mark,

I spoke with Joel recently. I have been hearing from people about him for some time; he spreads the word well. He told me he was in Cuba and became very sick. He went to an emergency room and the hospital personnel asked him if he had any pre-existing conditions. He told them he had hep C. They checked him for it and could not find it.

When he returned home, he went to a university in Michigan and had extensive blood work done. They told him he had no trace of hepatitis C. Joel told me he had been doing some herbal items for nine months and then started my program. About 45 days later, he tested negative for hepatitis C.

Lloyd

## Several Months and Doing Much Better

Dear Lloyd,

This is just a quick note of thanks for being there. After several months on your program, my fever has gone away, my diabetes has gone away, my energy level has improved, and my liver panels have been reduced significantly. I wish I had found your program back in August 2000 when my numbers were really high. I am not healed yet, but I know I am on my way. My AST went from 112 to 60 and my ALT went from 201 to 106. Thanks for everything, Lloyd!

Sincerely,<br>Tommy

## Hep C As Complex As AIDS

Lloyd,

I did buy your book a couple weeks ago. If all the bold print stuff about what you took was condensed to a couple of pages, that would be a big help, I think.

I will bring it to my doctor to see what he thinks. I feel fine and have little or no symptoms. My ALT is only slightly elevated. I am sure you get lots of email every day. One question, since everybody is different, what is good for one goose might be too little or too much for the other goose? Thanks for the info.

All the best in peace,<br>Chuck

Hi Chuck,

You are right about condensing the remedy into a one-page, easy-to-understand list. My new edition will have it.

You may show it to your doctor, but most conventional doctors are negative about this program. Not all of them. People who do what is in my book tend to get well. It is a very good immune system boost, and that is the main issue that needs to be addressed with hepatitis C. Your doctor will disagree.

As far as geese go, your doctor would prescribe interferon in the same amount regardless of which goose you were. We are dealing with a very complex virus, one that is almost as complex as the AIDS virus.

In good health,<br>Lloyd

## Interferon Worse than Rat Poison

Dear Lloyd,

Oh boy, pills too big to swallow, the tea tastes yukky. And just think, their alternative interferon is worse than rat poison. You know, I think getting well or getting anything you want in life takes really wanting it. That means believing in yourself and fighting for it. It means focus and some real drive. I think a large part of someone getting well is their own will and determination. I know I play the major role in whether I get well or not. You know, I have been doing some reading lately, and they have done some studies on the type of people that survive these kinds of things.

The ones with the best statistics are the fighters. The second best statistics belong to those who just ignore it, and the ones who succumb are most often the ones who complain and whine and feel sorry for themselves.

In case I haven't told you this before, you have already helped me a lot. I used to be in the first category. I fought and studied and was on a herbal/glandular type program. Then I found out about thymus and was even half-heartedly taking it. I did know, somehow, that the thymus I had was poor quality. My numbers went down anyway. I started feeling much better and then quit. I went into a big protest and decided to completely ignore it. But after one year, I started feeling kind of bad again.

I happened to see your book on the Internet and I bought and read it. I knew immediately that you had completed the medical research I had started. I knew your research was more thorough than mine, and I knew you were well. You finished what I started. And you were well.

When I got the products you recommended, I could tell instantly the difference in the quality between them and what I was on before. The products, coupled with the drive you have, which was so evident in your book, pushed me back into category one. I had received the inspiration I needed to get back into participating in my own recovery. It restored my willingness to fight back. I knew in my heart that this program had what my previous one was missing, and I knew my bad attitude was not helping anything. So for me, this all fits. Maybe those people who don't pull themselves up by the bootstraps and fight to get well just aren't ready to get well yet. It can be a tricky, boot tough, and mysterious world, can't it? To quote a brilliant man,

"Only the real tigers survive, and sometimes even they have a hard time at it."

Now, in less than a week, the difference in the way I feel is like night and day. I had been experiencing light headaches and muscle pains on-and-off all day, and now I don't even notice it anymore. Yesterday I realized I had been completely pain-free all day.

I also thought I had gained 5 pounds or so over the winter because my jeans weren't fitting anymore. I was gonna drag myself to the gym, even though I didn't feel that great. It was all bloat. Now my jeans fit, my shoes are comfortable again with thick socks on, and my face is back to normal. It had been getting kind of puffy, and I just thought I had put on some weight. Today I am going to the gym because I want to. Post this. Someone may need to read it.

Barry

## Japanese Client Has Never Seen Such Dramatic Improvement

Dear Mr. Wright,

My father has been under the conventional therapy of IV infusion of various vitamins, placenta–the standard protocol for hepatitis patients. In addition, he has been taking Chinese herbs: powdered drugs that are prescription drugs in Japan (ingredients include bupleurum, licorice, white peony root, etc.). These cover some of your protocol.

Since his blood test worsened in March, and he was not feeling well, I turned to a Japanese web site for alternative medicine.

From around 6/25, Natcell Thymus was added to his protocol and from around 7/1 to 7/7 some Amazon herbs against tumor (cat's claw, pau d'arco, graviola, etc.), as well as picao preto, boldo, erva tostao, etc.

His blood test of 7/24 (only about a month after the Natcell Thymus) showed amazing result! His ALB became normal, alpha 1G became normal, A/G ratio improved from 1.4 to 1.6. His AST got normal (from 48 to 38), ALT stayed normal, gamma GT came down (from 393 to 293). Hyalruronic acid came down (from 318 to 158) also!

As far as I know from this data of this year, I have never seen this dramatic improvement in so many parameters like this!

Again, thank you very much for your info. He is very hopeful now and we are both very much looking forward to the next blood test result and viral count test.

Atsuko<br>Japan

## Even In India, There Is a Will And a Way
## A Story From Lloyd

Alex began participating in a portion of my program on 9/27/2000. At the time he did not have a baseline viral load. His AST was 140 and ALT 226.

Over the months, he ordered a lot of Natcell Thymus and most of the major components of my program. He then traveled to India and took the frozen thymus with him to a place where there is little electricity or dry ice. Yet, he still managed to keep it frozen the whole time. While not doing the entire program, he did diligently participate in a good deal of it.

After approximately eight months Alex informed me that he no longer felt any symptoms. His ALT and AST are in the normal range and his viral load is 138,000. He expressed a need to cut back due to financial concerns, since he is in the normal range and no longer felt sick. He's come a long way and I congratulate him on his persistence.

Lloyd

## AST Dropped 100 Points In One Month
## Phone call from "Bobby" in Florida

"Bobby" was very happy to inform me that his ALT and AST have dropped dramatically.

In December his AST (SGTP) was 234 and his ALT (SGOT) 166.

By February his AST (SGTP) was 91 and his ALT (SGOT) 80.

This is after being on part of my program for one month, including Natcell Thymus.

Lloyd

## So Much Energy I Can't Stop

Dear Lloyd:

Just wanted to let you know that I feel so much better after one month of your treatment. I am so excited, and I have so much energy I cannot get normal sleep. It is nice to have my life back. I give the Lord the credit because He helped me find your web site.

Today we had an appointment at the transplant center. They put me through the stress test, breath test, echo, etc. The results were staggering compared to last November. Thank the Lord they did not do a viral load test. My load was 850,000 in November. Now it is surely much lower. I am afraid they will throw me out of the transplant center when I have to fess up and tell them what is making the difference.

Thanks,<br>Esther S.

## Cleared Up My Rash, Too!

Hi Lloyd,

It was good talking to you yesterday. You can't imagine how nice it is to talk to a real, knowledgeable person about something that I've been in the dark about for so many years. One day you will no doubt have to hire a person to answer your phone, but I am very pleased to have the privilege of working with you personally.

It has been just over three weeks since I started your program, and I'm doing almost everything you suggest. I have left out one of the herbs, but I'm even drinking the fairly disgusting mushroom tea! Thus far, it is difficult to tell if I have made much progress, since I am still having some trouble sleeping, but do you want to know about one significant change?

Approximately fourteen years ago, I developed a rash in a specific area of my body. This specific area doesn't often see daylight, and I have treated it with all manner of medications, topically and internally. It was very persistent and only responded to a strong fungal cream that I get from my vet for the dog's ears. This temporary relief would last one to three days.

So, in this short period of time, the rash has for the most part gone! I say most part because there is indeed scarring after so many years and a bit of redness persists, but no itching and weeping! This must indeed be a result of the combination of herbs and vitamins that I have recently introduced to my poor, needy body.

Thank you Lloyd!
Mitchell

## Developing A Taste for Nutrition

Lloyd,

I re-did the tea the way you said. Thanks bud, you are right. And when you put it that way, I'll swallow poo on a stick if it'll work. Besides, I have never felt sooooo good since I found you.

Hey, you were right about the glandular thymus. Whoa, what a difference, much stronger. Still trying to get up the dough for the Natcell, but feel good; my mind is a lot clearer and I'm not misplacing stuff around the house anymore. I'm able to keep up chores around here without trying to fall asleep on my feet.

So YOU ARE THE BOSS! I WILL LISTEN AND LEARN.

Stay healthy and God bless,
Sue

## ALT & AST Lowest In 5 Years–Phone conversation

On September 14, 2000, a man who had purchased *Triumph Over Hepatitis C* the previous February called me to share his recent blood test with me. He told me his doctor had been his friend all his life. Five years ago, his doctor told him to use interferon, as he was diagnosed with hepatitis C and cirrhosis. The man refused.

When he called me, he was quite happy and had a very deep sense of emotional appreciation. He told me his ALT and AST were lower than they had been over the last 5 years.

Before reading *Triumph Over Hepatitis C:*

| Date | AST | ALT | GGT |
|------|-----|-----|-----|
| 01/28/00 | 129 | 231 | 221 |

After reading *Triumph Over Hepatitis C:*

| Date | AST | ALT | GGT |
|------|-----|-----|-----|
| 08/26/00 | 36 | 72 | 148 |

This man did not do the entire program, but he used most of the recommended teas and many of the supplements. After seeing these results, he immediately ordered the live cell thymus.

To receive this wonderful report from a man with cirrhosis was a spectacular event. I have been professing that milk thistle tea and other items in my remedy can reverse cirrhosis. His doctor wanted to perform another biopsy to check the cirrhosis, but he refused.

His blood tests are on file.

Lloyd

## Not As Fatigued As Two Weeks Ago

Hey, Lloyd,

The taste of the live cell thymus is becoming more tolerable. The pain in my side has been gone now for two weeks, and I am not as fatigued as I was just two weeks ago. I have been taking all the supplements suggested in your book except the alfalfa (allergy) for six weeks now.

Reggie

## So Afraid of the Meds

Dear Lloyd,

I have a lot of faith in God, but to tell you the truth, when the doctors said, "You have hepatitis C," in my mind I thought I was dying, and I would be dead in a few days.

I believe in miracles. My ALT count was 40 and it went lower. I know you know the feeling of wondering every day, "Well, is the pain going to come again today, but then faith steps in and says NO."

I have not taken the meds the doctors want me to. I am so afraid of them that I am only taking the herbs, milk thistle, and the formula that contains thymus.

Thank you for all of your information and help. With people like you, life is still with us. Keep me in your prayers and you are in mine. Lets beat this thing, and help others beat it also with strong faith and nature.

Your friend,
Georgianna

## Started Feeling Better Within A Week

Lloyd,

I know hep C can be deadly, and after the look on my MD's face when he told me I should go ahead with the interferon, I should be pretty upset. Well, I am not upset, and don't plan on getting upset. In fact, I am looking forward to seeing the look on the doc's face while I am explaining why my next blood work shows such a great improvement.

A day or two after I found out the hep C was not going to stay inactive, a very good friend sent me to your web site. I got your book and studied it during the weekend. It wasn't long before I knew your treatment was the way to go. I ordered some of the products and within the first week, I started feeling better, so much better that I went off my Claritin D, Prilosec, Cardura, Orphenadrine, and Wellbutrin.

I hadn't started the teas yet, and soon I began seeing dark urine and the strong odor returned. As I write, I am looking out the window for the truck bringing more thymus, and my mailbox for the other goodies I ordered.

Thanks again,<br>Henry

## Back to Interferon?  Maybe NEVER!

Dear Lloyd,

I started on alpha lipoic acid and vitamin C back in early December, along with a few other vitamins and natural products. As you may recall, I started on your program just under two weeks ago.

I had my doctor draw some blood Monday, and I got the results today: ALT 59, AST 35. The last numbers I remember were 199 and 83 respectively. I'm sure the alpha lipoic and vitamin C were already working to bring these numbers down, but they didn't seem to help the way I was feeling.

I honestly can't say how long it's been since I've felt this good physically. Also, my color is improving, which was disturbing me greatly. I'm recently divorced, and I have more than a healthy dose of vanity.

Also, I was hoping you could give me more recommendations on diet. I'm avoiding all the things you say to in your book, and I gave up alcohol and drugs many years ago. My one remaining "vice" is coffee, which I hate to even think about letting go of, but I also like living. How bad is caffeine on the liver and immune system?

It's very early about using your program, but I'm extremely optimistic about this now and I'm not stressing out daily about when I'm going to start back on interferon, maybe NEVER!

Thanks for everything.<br>Carl

## Has Boycotted Pharmaceuticals

Dear Lloyd,

Wow, I just finished reading your book in one sitting, and I'm so excited. We are definitely kindred souls. I entirely share your view about the medical profession and have boycotted pharmaceuticals for some time now.

I've known I've had hep C since 1991, but I have probably had it for over 30 years, since I had acute hep B after a short but very stupid flirtation with drugs back in my 20's. I've been doing many of the herbs and lifestyle practices you recommend, but clearly not in the ultra-high dosages you recommend. I definitely will place an order. I'm sending a contribution via check, too.

God Bless, Judy<br>Fairfax, VA

## It's the Same in Switzerland

Dear Lloyd,

I read your book *Triumph Over Hepatitis C* two times cover-to-cover. I can't thank you enough for the wonderful job you have done, and would like to congratulate you on your success over hepatitis C.

I'm a 34-year-old woman from Switzerland suffering from chronic hepatitis C for over 10 years, and have been recommended to start Interferon treatment immediately. Because of my past experiences with medical doctors in Switzerland and the States (they are all the same), I have decided to do some research by myself.

I have come to the conclusion that I will NOT undergo any Interferon treatment, and that I'll combat this disease the natural way, hopefully with your help.

Siri

## Taking My Own Health Under Control

Dear Lloyd,

Thanks for answering me. When I read your information, it was like my whole world opened up. By the way, my doctors say that herbal meds do not work. I am taking my own health under control. I need help.

Jo Anne

## Conventional Medicine Really Put Me Off

Hello again:

I just wanted to write again and say that I have been reading more of your site. I must say that if you really are cured with no detectable virus, then that is the best news I have ever heard in my life.

Conventional medicine really put me off and I am determined to do exactly the same as you have. Now I have faith. Somewhere inside me I thought it must be possible to do, but now you seem to be proof of that.

One of my life goals is to do exactly what you have done and that is to educate people with this disease and help them be cured. I am currently living in L.A., but I will be going home to Australia in July. Once I am cured (positive thinking), I will start with the people in the hep C clinic at the depressing hospital, which of course I have been part of.

If you have any time, you could maybe reply to my emails with more words of wisdom and encouragement, because lately I have been having a really hard time dealing with it. But I am feeling a lot better since I read your site, so thank you for that. If you don't have time, I understand.

With love from the happy reader,<br>
Chris

## Down to Earth and Easy to Follow

Dear Lloyd,

I received the book the other day and started reading it immediately. I love the way it's written, so down to earth and easy to follow. Your sense of humor's not too shabby either!

I want to get started so badly, but a little at a time. Financially, well, let's just say I'm being very positive. I start a new job Monday at a greenhouse. I love working outside with the earth and getting dirty. Plants and veggies are something I know about, so I'm looking forward to this new endeavor.

My 77-year-old mom has been such a sweetheart. She thinks she's 20 and still acts like it. She is a garage sale, flea market addict. She came over here Saturday morning with a brand new juicer still in the box. She paid $10 for it. Brought me fresh beets, carrots, spinach, broccoli, you name it. She's so cute. She also bought me two bottles of milk thistle. So I'm on my way!

I still smoke. I know anything I do with herbs will just be depleted, so I'm working on that. Say a prayer for me.

Your friend,
Deb

## Want to Rid Myself of This Before It Happens

Dear Mr. Wright,

Thank you for responding so quickly. I'm very anxious to get started on your program. I'm not sick yet and would like to rid myself of this before it happens. Thanks again.

Joni

## For So Many Years, Nobody Understood

Dearest Lloyd,

Hi and hello. I am glad to talk to somebody who understands what it is all about. For so many years, nobody understood what was going wrong. All the doctors said we worked too hard and had too much stress. That was the reason for my problem of feeling tired and so many depressions you could not understand. What a misery all these years. I know and feel that this is going to work because in the literature you can find some indications, but for the medical team THINKING about a problem is toooooooo much to ask, if you see what I mean.

Rita is drinking distilled water since we read about it in your book. She puts a bit of lemon in it, and it is fine to drink! We're going to start dandelion and licorice next week. Hoping to give you positive results. I cannot thank you enough.

Warm and kindest regards, Hilde
Belgium

## Thanks for Being Accessible

Thanks, Lloyd,

I did get two books, but no matter, 'cause I wanted to order one for my best friend who is also in the battle. I feel much more positive about the route I want to take, thanks to you. I had a few good laughs while reading your book.

She feels the same way about doctors and interferon as I do, so your book will make a great gift. I'm sure I will have questions. Thanks again for making yourself so accessible.

Laurie

Hello Laurie,

You are fighting a war! That is the way I look at hep C. It is a war you can win if you use the right smart bombs. You made an excellent choice for a beginning. I'm here to help!

Thank you,<br>Lloyd

## Big Inspiration

Hey, Lloyd,

Thank you for sending me my herbs so promptly. I loved your book. You have been a big inspiration to me.

Thanks again,<br>Ron

## Surprising Results

Dear Lloyd,

After being on the program for 90 days, I had to go to my liver doctor to get approval for surgery on my knee.

They ran a blood panel, and the test results came back with normal liver enzyme levels of 47. Unfortunately, I have a genotype of 1a. I will continue the treatment and hope that the viral count that was over 8 million last fall will begin to drop. I would be interested in any new or additional therapy advances that become available. Thanks for helping us all (hep C positive) out there!

Marcille

## Gland Swelling Gone in Just Eight Days.
## Thank You From the Bottom of My Heart

Dear Lloyd,

I'd like to give you some feedback about my reaction to your program. So far, it's been nothing short of miraculous.

On 9/25/01, I was diagnosed with HCV. I had been feeling a little off for a couple years, but couldn't put my finger on the problem. Previously I hadn't been to a doctor for over 25 years. I had always felt great until then.

After returning from a vacation that involved heavy drinking, I felt terrible, and I had a feeling it was more than just a hangover. I scheduled a doctor's appointment and had numerous blood tests. That's how I found out. The doctor scheduled an ultrasound and referred me to a hepatologist. I went home, got on the web, and started studying the disease. I was shocked and scared. After the ultrasound, I went to the liver specialist who suggested a biopsy and then Rebetron combo therapy.

I wanted to try modification of my diet and the herb therapy I was reading about on the web, but he was not impressed. He ordered a genotype test and set a follow-up appointment that's coming up on 11/15/01.

It was time for me to make some important decisions. My health situation was severely affecting the quality of my life. I was tired. I had to nap 2 to 3 times a day. I could feel my liver almost like heartburn all the time. I had terrible memory problems and difficulty concentrating. At this point, I was reading every book I could get my hands on and spending hours on the web gathering information and perspectives. The list of side effects associated with interferon scared me.

I was hoping to find a different, more credible course of action. I changed my diet: nothing but organic foods, no caffeine, no alcohol, no aspirin, and I bought a vegetable juicer and organic cookbooks. My theory is that I'll only put things in my body that are good for my liver and immune system and nothing else, to give my liver the chance to rest and regenerate. I've always worked out, but I've become more serious, 5 days a week, even if I'm tired.

I bought the herbs I read about and started taking them. After about 10 days I felt better. One of the books I read was yours. I got on your web site and was intrigued that you had cleared yourself of the virus. On 10/22/01 I called you against the advice of my mother, a nurse and my doctor who wants me to start interferon/Ribavirin therapy. We spoke and I was encouraged by your enthusiasm and my fear of the side effects of interferon, so I decided to try it for the 18-month interval. I ordered a three-month supply including Natcell Thymus and Natcell Liver, which is expensive.

However, I have no prescription drug coverage with my health insurance and surmised after consultation with my doctor that your program for me is about the same price as the regular drug combo therapy. Combine that with the fact that if it worked, it would be abundantly less expensive because I could keep working through the treatment. With my diet modifications and herbal supplementation I felt better, but my health situation was still severely affecting the quality of my life.

I started your program 10/24/01 and felt better every single day. For the last year and a half, the lymph glands on the sides of my neck have been swollen like walnuts. On the eighth day when I woke up in the morning, the swelling was GONE! I am stunned, I feel better than I have in two years, after only EIGHT DAYS on your program! My memory's back, I have no difficulty concentrating, and I can work a full day without getting tired. I almost feel like I'm not sick anymore; I can't wait to test my blood again in 3 months!

I feel that the Natcell was the key, as I received it first and have only used the supplements four of the eight days. After feeling the immediate affect of assisting my thymus gland and assisting my liver regenerate with the Natcell products, I also want to assist my adrenal gland, which I'm sure has been weakened trying to fight this disease during its incubation period. I have decided to incorporate the Natcell Adrenal and ordered it today.

About your line of supplements, after reading your book and others, I went to the vitamin store and purchased some of the supplements recommended. After I received your package, I planned to finish what I had already purchased, then start with yours. However, after comparing products I literally looked at what I had bought at the vitamin store as junk. The ingredients and manufacturing procedures of your products were superior to what I already had. Your supplements, which are targeted and tailored for enhancement of the immune system and support of the liver, are just what I am looking for.

In general, as I said, I am stunned. I feel tremendously lucky that I found your web site and very thankful that you took the time to answer my questions. Had I not talked with you when I did, I most likely would be getting ready to start my combo therapy in 2 weeks. When you're sick and told you have a very serious disease with a very small chance for a cure and you can feel it taking over your body, you'd give anything for your health back. Your program has given me so much hope for the future. Thank you from the bottom of my heart. I'll keep you informed, as my new blood tests will be taken in 3 months.

Sincerely,
Bob

## Sneak In Good Anti-Depressants

Dear Lloyd,

Hope you are doing well. Today I have a question for you: the thing is that my family doctor has put me on depression pills. Would that interfere in any way with the other ingredients you have suggested to me, even if they are natural products? I would very much like to start with the recipe you have given me.

Thanks,
Francine

Dear Francine,

What kind of depression pills? You start on my program and you won't be depressed any more. You will have cause to celebrate each day for the rest of your life. We can also sneak in some good natural anti-depressants.

Lloyd

### Terrific Results!  A Story From Lloyd

On August 20, 2000, a 65-year-old male (I'll call K.M.) began my program with a viral load of greater than 800,000 and elevated AST and ALT. After 2 1/2 months on my program, his AST and ALT are normal and his viral load has dropped to 338.000.

# THREE

## PANDORA'S BOX

Becoming triumphant over hepatitis C isn't just about overcoming an illness, as you can see from the letters in this chapter. Discovering you have hepatitis C opens up a whole can of worms, which reminds me of the fable of Pandora's Box, a story that is similar to the story of Adam and Eve and the forbidden fruit.

According to Greek mythology, Pandora was the first woman on earth. She was created from earth and water by the god Vulcan (who, by the way, is not Mr. Spock from "Star Trek"). The gods and goddesses bestowed her with many attributes, and thus she was named Pandora, meaning "all-gift."

When Pandora was presented to the god Epimetheus, she brought with her a box that the other gods had told her never to open. But her curiosity was too strong and she finally raised the lid. All the vices and sins, diseases and troubles in the world at once flew out of the box. Pandora shut the lid quickly, but all except one thing had escaped, and that one thing was HOPE, the only item left to console humans.

In the following letters, my clients express, and often anguish over, the many issues that crop up after they open up their own personal "Pandora's Box" and discover they have hepatitis C. But the strength of their human spirit prevails, as they are guided by the hope they can conquer this illness.

## Lloyd Missed the Indianapolis 500 and it Was Worth It!

Tony C. called me on Memorial Day and told me he was going to be in my area. He asked if he could meet with me to pick up his products so he could avoid the shipping charges.

Tony began my program on March 29, 2001. At first I was upset that I was going to miss half of the Indianapolis 500, and I hadn't had a day off for 18 months. However, after the first few moments of speaking with this man, I felt very much rewarded.

Tony informed me that he didn't have the money to do this health regimen, so he went to the company he worked for and asked if he could take money out of his retirement fund to participate in my program. He told me his boss urged him not to do it, but to keep that money for his family for when he was gone. At the time, Tony was quite sick and had taken leave from work because he could no longer function in his position.

On Memorial Day weekend, I felt so good about this man. He related to me how he had gone from being unable to work at all to working full time and feeling very healthy. He looked very healthy. He explained to me his thinking: What good would his money do for his family without him? He said to me that working was the best thing he could do for both his employer and his family; now he is happily doing just that.

He described to me how he wrestled with the disease: the fatigue and the flu-like symptoms. He shared with me in detail the effort of going to a shopping mall with his family and having to sit down on the floor because he simply could not continue to stand.

Listening as Tony described his condition and the changes he experienced in the first few months brought back to me memories of my own story when I was in exactly the same dilemma. I'm very happy I took time out to go meet with this man. The feelings he shared with me were heart-warming. I love him as I would a brother. He caused me to see that missing a sports event on T.V. is of little importance. Rather, to have a true human experience with someone in person is far more enlightening than anything.

Lloyd

## This Can Be a Lonely Disease

Lloyd,

How awesome you responded so quickly! Thank you! Of course, you may feel free to post my email on the message board. I have read the messages, and they have been so informative and helpful. It helps so much to know we are not alone. This can really be a lonely disease, as I'm sure you know.

My husband is reading your book and likes what he is hearing. He is a wonderful man, but I'm afraid he is now a food addict. He gave up all his other addictions to nicotine, alcohol, and drugs of various hallucinogenic properties. Now he loves his coffee with cream, sugar, pies, and meat! I, on the other hand, am a recovering anorexic, compulsive exerciser! What a pair we make, huh?

Anyway, I think the idea of giving up his favorite foods is scary to him. If he only knew how wonderful he would feel if he did! Even though he is off the interferon, he is still experiencing extreme fatigue, nausea, headaches, and skin rashes, among other things.

We have a three-year-old daughter. She is beautiful, bright, and a ball of wild energy. She can't understand why her daddy can't play with her very much, why he is tired all the time, and why he doesn't feel good.

I can buy all of the products you suggest, but I can't force him to do what he is not willing to do, you know? I will support him all I can. This has been so hard on all of us. I just want his to get better.

Thanks for being a sounding board for me!

Holly

Dear Holly,

I have encountered many who feel that only their doctor knows best, but most people who do the interferon realize that they have to do this differently. Most of my clients have done interferon and love my program. It makes you feel human again, and at the same time you get well.

Lloyd

## I Actually Cooked For Myself

Dear Lloyd,

Just a note to let you know I actually cooked for myself this week. I even made a big pot of vegetable stew.

AND I can drive again. Today is such a beautiful day here in Tucson, the sun shining, not a cloud in the sky, and it's almost 70 degrees. Since it's Sunday, there's not so much traffic, and I was feeling clear-headed, so away I went. My little F150 and ME took a ride. I drove for 20 miles. I haven't even driven 20 blocks in the last few months.

I actually feel as though I've just gotten out of jail! This is all because of the hope and guidance you have given to me.

Thank you, my friend,
Nancy

## Without the BS of Conventional Medicine

Dear Lloyd!

Well you said not to get my hopes up regarding the blood work and I didn't, but here we go. With just two months of seriously taking the remedies, my homeopath has prescribed doing your program. With only one order of the frozen thymus, plus all your other good stuff, the results look like this:

| Date | AST | ALT | GGT |
|------|-----|-----|-----|
| 10/13/2000 | 205 | 211 | 66 |
| 1/11/2001 | 140 | 165 | 55 |

I have to say while it's not perfect (yet), I'm going to get there. I didn't start seeing my new doc until December, and I didn't really start everything on your list (in fact I still don't take everything) because my homeopath doesn't want me to overload the liver.

The only other concern we are working on now is the iron, which, although it has gone from 263 to 242, still stinks. Just today I went to see a hematologist, and of course, he requested blood work to see if it is a genetic disorder. You're right; anyone with MD attached to their name should be avoided at all costs. The consultation was depressing to say the least.

Now I have to go back to him in 2 weeks to discuss phlebotomies. But I might just flee and find someone else, which is pretty difficult around here. You can't just get a lab to take this "tainted blood." You have to literally go underground to find someone to do this. I've been tempted to do like the Romans–very week just lie bleeding in a hot tub, then have someone call EMS and let them patch up my wrists, and try to stay out of a mental institutions, but I'm sure the insurance company would wonder after a while.

So, that being said, I think I'm on the right track. If I have to smoozle up with this MD just to get the iron out, I'll do it. My homeopath feels that the iron has to go before we can even think about eradicating this gosh-darn virus.

So that's it in a nutshell. If you need me to send you these labs, just let me know. I'd rather send them when the results are  great and over, but they're here for you if you need them to help prove that it can be done without all the BS of conventional medicine.

Take care,
Vernon


## I Didn't Realize How Sick I'd Been Until I Began To Feel Better

Dear Lloyd,
The doctor ordered a metabolic panel to monitor use of Celebrex. My ALT has dropped significantly, from 219 to 69 and my AST from 111 to 94. That's only after two months on your program. I didn't realize how sick I've been for the last 12-15 years until I started to feel better.

Thank you, Ellie

## Encounters Stigma and Prejudice from Doc

Hi There,

I wanted you to know I read your book and found it very useful. My situation is that I did try the interferon A and Ribavirin program. My liver enzymes are normal, but I still have the virus. My last viral load was 770,000, much too high for me, even though this is still considered low. I want it to be 0000!

My liver biopsy showed no damage to my liver, only slight inflammation. Apparently, the doctors think this was something that I just got. That was one year ago.

I also have the same opinion of the medical field as you. The doctors were horrible. They were insistent that I was either a drug addict or prostitute. The doctor who monitored me during the interferon/Ribavirin treatment (gastroenterologist) made me feel like I was going to die soon. She never read me my records and was always saying things like maybe I was a Stage 1 or Stage 2 case. When I asked her how many stages are there, her response was "three!"

At the end, when I tried to find out exactly what my numbers were, she was so harsh she brought me to tears. I was definitely dying. It took me a year to get over it. Anyway, that's past, and with your help I can get on the right program.

Looking forward to hearing from you!

Thanks again,
Sheila

## THOUGHT IT WAS TERMINAL

Dear Lloyd, Hello and thank you. Please tell me more about overcoming hep C. I thought I had a terminal disease.

Randy

## V.A. NOT HELPING VIETMAN VET

Dear Lloyd,

My husband is a Vietnam vet, and he has been diagnosed with hep B for years. The V.A. (Veterans Administration) told him over a year ago that he no longer has hep B but now has hep C. He was supposed to have a biopsy over 6 months ago, but they keep canceling and rescheduling. The last 3 or 4 months his stomach has started to bloat. It is very bad now. He is skinny down to the bone. He looks like a concentration camp victim, even though he says he feels good and he has a good appetite. But I am very worried.

The V.A. doesn't seem to be doing anything (not seem to be, they haven't). Can you give me some advice, please? If he waits until June for the next appointment, I am afraid he will be dead!

Most sincerely,
Lori

### What a Shock!

Dear Lloyd,

I have just been diagnosed with HCV. What a shock! I am a personal trainer and extremely healthy. But I used injectable street drugs for a short time when I was 17, and that is where they are saying it came from. My ex-husband has also been diagnosed. He did drugs too. Of course, I have been reading and researching in every spare minute, and your book has caught my attention over everything else.

THANK YOU,
Jhan

## We Want to Survive This

Dear Lloyd,

Hello. We are a couple in Van Nuys, California, who are hep C carriers. We have been together for the past 30 years and contracted the virus through IV use when we were in our 20s. Both of us have had two liver biopsies, a liver scan and basically nothing else, including any type of information regarding symptoms or treatments from our liver specialist at UCLA.

We both have been experiencing symptoms for quite a while, my wife more than I, until recently. Stress has us both going through "C" hell. A month ago, I threw up 1/4 glass of bile, and then a few days ago I had an episode that scared the hell out of me. My fingertips in my left hand went cold and at the same time my upper left quadrant and around my spleen felt like I had hot coals burning.

I went to the emergency room. I filled out the questionnaire, listed hep C, and was seen by a Dr. Caldron. After listing all my symptoms, he said that he believed they the result of the hep C virus, and he went on to enlighten me as to all the symptoms and possible remedies in the real world of "C". He told me he could prescribe medicines, but that he thought I should see a man named Steve at a pharmacy in Santa Monica. I went to see Steve, he handed me your book, and he suggested I start with Hepastat and Hepata Trope.

I am a working husband in very competitive selling of services. My wife cares for a large and hectic household. Our stress levels are always very high. We have two grandchildren, two daughters and a son, and they all live with us.

We have read your book and are excited about the potential of finding a way to cope with this disease. We both would like to ask you a thousand questions. We want to survive this since we both have the virus and we have a large family that solely relies on me for at least 80% of everything.

Roger

## Had Hep C Since Age 4, and No Insurance

Hello, Lloyd,

I have hep C, and I recently went onto your web site and read your testimony and the testimony of others about how these herbs helped them. I am intrigued about how you are free of hep C after taking these herbs.

I'm 24 years old, and I've been diagnosed since 1997, but I believe that I've been infected since I was little. I got sick when I was 4 years old with anemia and hepatitis. I believe it was hep A. I received blood transfusions, and this was back in the early 80s when they didn't test the blood for hepatitis.

My hep C is not chronic or acute; it is just there. I've been to the doctor, and they have told me that my liver levels are going up. I have no insurance. When my family found out that I had hep C, they were devastated because they didn't think that I was going to be sick again. They've been trying to give me different remedies from our country.

Please give me some advice on what herbs to take, especially thymus that I read about. Thank you for your time.

Lila

Dear Lila,

What country do you live in? I can deliver my products to most countries. Even if you do not have symptoms, and even if your doctors tell you that everything is fine, you need to be doing things to stop the virus. Alternative medicine is new to the doctors, and they do not have any idea of what they speak. You will be just fine, but you need to do certain things for the rest of your life.

Milk thistle is one of the things you need to use. Just know that it must become part of your life. Take the tea from milk thistle seeds, the capsules, 400 mg. 3 times a day. Also, the following: lipoic acid, 200 mg. 3 times per day; selenium 400 mcgs per day; and, dandelion root tea, several cups per day, afternoon and evening. Properly prepared aloe, 4 oz. 3 times per day or more. These are things that should become as regular as eating. Natcell Thymus is also very good and can help put an end to the virus. The other items in my book will also help you put an end to this condition.

In good health,<br>Lloyd

## Airline Pilot Given Lots of Hope

Dear Lloyd,

What an awesome book! You should go on tour and start speaking to people to get the word out even more and to promote what you have discovered. Throw pie at those wacky doctors that are out there.

Anyway, I was diagnosed with HCV a year ago. I tried the combo therapy for a week and knew it was not for me. It was almost impossible to do the therapy, as I am a pilot for a major airline. I had surgery for a deviated septum about 10 years ago, and I suspect that's where I contracted the virus. Or it could have been a routine cleaning of the teeth at the dentist's office.

Again, I really appreciate your book and it has really opened my eyes and given me lots of hope at ending this dreaded disease.

Sincerely,
Mike

## Tenacity and Determination

Dear Lloyd:

May I say from the outset what an outstanding web site and wonderful information you have. I congratulate you for your tenacity and determination to overcome your challenge of hepatitis C.

I congratulate you even more for sharing the information you have gathered, so that others will find new hope in the alternative medicines you describe. Thank you for this gift on behalf of so many others.

Heino in Ontario, Canada

## Ready to Try Anything

Dear Mr. Wright,

I recently found out my brother was dying in the hospital from complications with the hepatitis C virus. I was searching the net and came across your book.

My brother is 46 years old, married, with 3 children. He had received a transfusion due to a great loss of blood from a hockey accident over 20 years ago. His liver is only 10% functional. He had a tumor on his kidney and he also had edema. Needless to say, he is in terrible shape. He was in a coma and on life-support from April 24 to April 29.

The liver specialist said they are doing all they can do for him, which does not seem to be very much. His breathing is very poor and he is bed-ridden. His case seems pretty hopeless and we want to try anything.

We were considering taking him to the CHIPSA clinic in Tijuana to get alternative treatments, but the doctor said he would not survive the trip, even in an air ambulance.

I spoke to my sister-in-law a few minutes ago, and she said that my brother now has kidney failure. Things do not look good at all. We really need help and will appreciate any advice you can give.

By the way, I am ordering a copy of your book and sending it to her today.

Sincerely,<br>Ron

Dear Ron,

This is a difficult situation. There are live peptides that can help end stage situations of this nature. I have seen people use them. They are expensive and can work wonders. I wish I could have met you a year earlier, and then the success rate would be better.

If I can be of further assistance, I am here.

Lloyd

## We Are Just Desperate

Hello,

Thanks so much for all of your insight and knowledge. My mother was diagnosed with HCV. She was told it is likely she has had it for roughly 27 years. She used to drink wine, and her doctor told her that she already has cirrhosis of the liver. However, he would like to confirm it via a liver biopsy. She is reluctant to do this and would like to try your treatment before going further with her physician. They make her outcome seem very bleak and quite morbid. She is 47 with 5 children, three still in school.

As I am sure you are already aware, this has turned our lives upside down and you bring quite a bit of hope to us. I read all of the survival stories from those that opted for your treatment. However, I am curious what the success stats are compared to those it does not work for. We are all trying to deal with this as realistically as possible, and your site gave us great hope. However, as I realize there are no guarantees, I do not want false hope either. Please let me know your thoughts, and I apologize for being so blunt and appearing "pushy," but we are just desperate. Thanks so very much.

Michelle

Dear Michelle,

Forty-seven is young and there is time for you to reverse this condition. During my research when writing *Triumph*

94

*Over Hepatitis C*, I encountered tremendous knowledge relating to reversing cirrhosis. I have now seen it with my own eyes in about 25 of my clients. It takes time and persistence. Of all the people who have done my entire program with persistence, only one person, a mother of ten, has not responded after one year. She is the only person I know of that actually did everything I did and had it fail. There are numerous reasons for it, but she is the only one.

Many start and never finish, many like to play chemistry set and do their own thing. I do not consider them failures because they did not do as I did. People who do what I did tend to get well.

In good health,<br>
Lloyd

## Preserve Your Sense of Humor

Dear Lloyd,

Went home for lunch today and your book was in my mailbox. Would have gotten back to you sooner but I couldn't put it down. I have already read it and it was SOO funny. It is great to see that you could preserve your sense of humor during such a crisis. Keeping our sense of humor makes everything a little bit easier.

THANKS AGAIN AND IT WAS GOOD READING!

Alma

## Struggling With a Life Crisis

Hello:

What can I say, except I do appreciate your comments and concern. Even though I don't know you, I feel you understand my paranoia and lack of trust are not directed at your personally. I was a very healthy, active guy, and now I'm struggling with a life crisis. Please send any and all information you feel would be of benefit to me.

Les

## Your Book Gives Us Great Hope

Dear Lloyd,

I want to thank you for your great, important book. It's incredible what you've successfully endured. It gives all of us hep C+ people great hope.

I currently have hep C (12 million count, phase 3 liver, slightly elevated ALT and AST), but no symptoms. I have implemented some of your advice (raw eggs, artichokes, spinach, no bovine milk, low fat, Vitamin C, distilled water), and I plan to implement more with time (buckwheat, alfalfa and milk thistle are next). I get steady exercise (tennis 3 times/week) and actively try to reduce stress. Any other additional information would be greatly appreciated. Thank you very much.

Larry

## In A State of "Overwhelm"

Mr. Wright,

I have had hep C for some time now. My last blood test revealed 100,000 rate of replication (did I say that right?). The doctor stated that the lab tests don't go any higher, and he wants me to see a specialist, have a biopsy done, and he discussed the interferon therapy.

I DON'T have positive feelings about this drug, although she says 1/3 of all patients were "undetectable" for the virus after doing this therapy. I have been taking

Silimarin, Beta Carotene, Lecithin, B Complex and Vitamin C. Is this enough? I am in a state of overwhelm. Thank you for the hope you have given me.

Trudie

## This Really Gives People Hope

Dear Lloyd,

I have been diagnosed with hep C also. I had surgery 20 years ago for removal of a brain tumor and I contracted it thru a blood transfusion.

I bought your book and read it. Boy, were you ever thru a lot. I cannot even imagine what you have gone thru. I am seeing a hepatologist from Philadelphia. He is just following my liver enzymes. I have not had a biopsy as of yet. He does not want to do the biopsy until my enzymes go up to one and one-half times normal. I do get very fatigued very easily, and I have been experiencing joint and muscle pain. My doctor is not alarmed by this. I am 52 years of age, and I work as a nurse in a life care community, working out of the resident nurses' office.

Your book was written with a lot of humor, which I enjoyed. I read it in one evening. This really gives people hope. I just want to say thanks, and I hope that you continue to do well.

Sincerely,<br>Carol

## My Father Needs Hope. He is Giving Up

Dear Lloyd,

I just stumbled over your web site tonight. I'm not even sure why I am writing to you. My dad has hep C. He contracted it in 1989 from open-heart surgery. He is 75 years old. He has always been very active, and he was a famous country musician. Now he lies in bed very nauseous. I am very into natural medicine and have had him try lots of natural remedies. Milk thistle has worked a miracle on his liver.

He tried the thymus stuff, but said it made him more nauseous. We don't have a lot of money to keep him on all the herbs. He is still waiting for his settlement. I don't know what to do anymore. Is your book really true? My father needs hope. He is giving up. Can you give us any hope? We live in Canada.

Thanks,<br>Tyra

Dear Tyra,

Your dad needs to try the right kind of thymus; it makes all the difference in the world. Have him call me; I can help.

Lloyd

P.S. I sell your father's song about hep C on my web site.

## Teenage Son Got HCV as a Child

Lloyd,

Thank you for your book. I too have experienced the lack of knowledge and lack of concern in dealing with the doctors regarding HCV. I asked the last doctor what he would do if it were his son. He seemed dismayed but offered us no help.

My son has HCV. He is 17 years old and got it 8 years ago in an operation. Kyle still has the virus no matter what we try.

Keeping in mind Kyle is holding his own, he is a little tired and his eyes are a little jaundiced, but his enzymes are within the upper normal limits and he is not as sick as you were. Which of the tons of pills and gallons of tea and liver and thymus cells would you recommend? What is the least amount of stuff you believe will kill the virus?

Anxiously awaiting your recommendation. Thanks.

Suzanne

## Your Story Keeps Me Going

Hi there, Lloyd!

I ordered your book about one week ago and I actually called you as well. You called me back with a very touching, lovely, and inspiring message. Thank you very much because you brightened my day when I really needed it. I absolutely loved your book. It was so inspiring, frank, and hilarious. You have an excellent sense of humor that I completely understand.

The reason I am writing to you is because about 2 1/2 weeks ago my boyfriend was diagnosed with hep C. He believes he contracted it in 1982. He is feeling okay, he's just always tired, and it doesn't help that he is a workaholic.

He hasn't been to the doctor since he was diagnosed because he has been too busy (hence the girlfriend on the net researching and writing to you). I am almost thankful that he hasn't been yet, after reading what really goes on inside those hospital walls. He will go, though, to see what's up with his levels, his liver, etc.

We are very interested in buying many of the products that you offer. I think it's brilliant that you have created this service. Wow! You are really turning your experience into something that helps others! Isn't that what we are here for! I love it that you are handling it this way! Thanks for sharing your story. It really keeps me going. I need my man alive, ya know. Also, we are having a baby, and we all really need dad around, alive and healthy. Your web site has given me such a positive and optimistic attitude.

Once again, thank you so much.

Shaheen

## Your Book Gave Me a Reason to Hope

Dear Mr. Wright,

I was amazed at the generosity of a human being in this world filled with Man's inhumanity to Man. Thanks for trusting me and know that I am remitting payment for your book. I found it very truthful and hilarious! Your book brightened up my day and gave me a reason to hope along with my prayers.

I have been taking the milk thistle, dandelion, NADA, thymus and slippery elm. Yes, don't forget the licorice. I know that this is just a drop in the bucket, but money is fleeting as usual. I know you might relate to this. I always pray for you and your continued remission from this horrible disease. I am telling everyone of your generosity and of your remarkable recovery!

I really thank God for you and will relinquish your attention and not continue to babble. It's just so nice to have someone to identify with, even if you are thousands of miles away. Again, thanks and may God bless you and keep you strong and with such an amazing sense of humor in the face of such alarming odds.

Respectfully yours,<br>Ceila

## Light of Hope

Dear Lloyd,

Everything came through just fine. Thank you so much for your kindness and caring. You've given us the light of hope in what have been some very dismal days. We'll be in touch.

God bless and keep you,<br>Michael & Jaz

## No Idea How I Contracted This Disease

Dear Lloyd,

I received your book on Saturday. Thank you; it's very interesting. I read the whole thing in one sitting. We are in the process of getting an order together and will be back in touch soon.

For your information, we have no idea how my husband contracted this disease. He's had no blood transfusions or drug use. It's real mystery to us. However, he is a veteran.

Sincerely,<br>Julie

## Going From Intron A to Thymus

Dear Mr. Wright,

I am looking forward to reading your book, and I will contact you again around September when my husband will be off the Intron A, so we can purchase the live thymus extract we discussed. May you stay healthy and happy and may God's blessings be upon you for the help you are giving to so many others.

Sincerely,<br>
Iris & Brian

## I've Seen It All and More!

Dear Lloyd,

Just read your book! My regret is that I did not read it sooner. My husband is eleven months post-transplant and was just diagnosed with FCH.

I've seen it all and more, just as you describe the medical practice! His only hope, until I read your book, was to begin Rebetron (although he is not strong enough to start treatment), or hope for another transplant. (Mt. Sinai is the only center re-transplanting FCH).

Of course, he is not strong enough for this either. I really feel like I've just seen a science experiment go wrong. He received a 6-month prognosis after his move from ICU where he was received in guarded condition. All this was due to the resident allowing him to thrash in pain for 2 1/2 hours after a kidney biopsy.

Thanks for another hope, if not more! Just knowing someone else sees it from the same perspective is a great help!

Rhonda

## Hep C and Relationships

Dear Lloyd,

I just wanted to say thank you for sending the book and replying to my emails. I am so looking forward to reading it. I feel a great deal better after reading that most of your clients that are in relationships have not caught the virus through sex. I assume they don't wear protection all the time. After all it is a blood-borne disease, even though the doctors I saw today said it is in bodily fluids as well. That's the strange thing; everyone says something different.

I have had the virus for 12 years. I am now nearly 31, and I don't think it matters that I have had it for such a long time. I am still capable of being cured also.

I am on a mission to help people get well (as well as myself). I am so happy that I found your web site. You have no idea how much relief I feel. I have faith.

Bye for now,
K.

Dear Lloyd,

I think it is a wonderful thing you are doing, and it seems to me that this is your life purpose, as they say everything happens for a reason. I am grateful to have come across you. I will keep in touch and let you know of my progress, and keep up the amazing work.

Very grateful and happy,
K.

## Hope Your Book Sales Skyrocket

Hello again, Lloyd,

I've just finished reading your book. I tell you what, you almost literally went thru HELL. I'm sure glad you had the will and desire to do all the research that you have done to heal yourself, and I thank you for sharing it with my wife and I and the others who will read your book.

I hope your book sales skyrocket, because if this remedy worked for you and others since you, you damn sure deserve it.

Sincerely yours,
John

## Won't Go Alternative-Medicine Hopping, But He's Willing To Try This

Dear Mr. Wright,

First of all, thank you for this book and the hope it's given me.

My boyfriend Gary is 49 years old, and he had a motorcycle accident about 20 years ago. He's had 30 operations since the accident; the last one was around 1990-1991. In 1998, our doctor tested him for hep C, and he was told he had it and that it was dormant.

Gary went to the doctor's for allergies, and the nurse practitioner took tests to check on his hep C. They called later that week and said it was active. The nurse practitioner was pushing for the scientific route and told him to see a specialist, which we will, but we told him we were trying this route too.

Thank you sooooo much for your help. I really don't have anyone else to ask these questions to because Gary won't go alternative-medicine hopping, but he's willing to try this.

Leslie

## Please Tell Me Someone I Can Trust

To whom it may concern:

I'm a methadone patient, and aside from my 75-milligram daily dose, I'm drug-free and I do not drink alcoholic drinks. I have not used any heroin or any other injectable or otherwise illegal drugs in over 5 years.

I was informed about 4 years ago that I was hep C positive. I can tell from the pain (not terrible pain, but pain each day) and the hardness of my liver that I need HELP! I am really scared and have tried to rely on faith alone to get me thru. But, I am thinking that I am getting closer and closer to death, and I am afraid.

I am a medical patient at the clinic and they do have pamphlets about hep C, but I don't trust them. I've only seen a doctor twice for hepatitis. He sorta scared me, plus I don't understand him very well because of his Indian accent.

I am a husband and the father of 4 and my stepdaughter. I'm 38 years old. I can't stand thinking of leaving them, especially my 3-year-old baby girl. I know it would hurt her a lot, because I take care of her and my wife works. I love her deeply too. She is so wonderful to love me, a man with such a horrific past and so much wasted life. Would you PLEASE tell me someone I can trust to go for help?

Mike

Dear Mike,

I can help you! There is no need to pay a doctor to rip you off while you do this. There are minimal things one can do that stop the virus from doing serious damage. It is another thing to get rid of it. This is a minimum and works quite well for many symptoms and can stop or slow progression of the virus:

Milk thistle 400 mg 3 times per day
Lipoic acid 200 mg 3 times per day
Selenium 400 mcg per day
Dandelion root tea, 1 quart a per day

I am here if you need further info.

Lloyd

## Doctors Don't Tell You Very Much

Dear Lloyd,

I have been looking at your site, and I have read everything on it. I have found the message board very informative. It's good to hear people with the same problems talk so positive and hear their hope for success over this virus.

I called your number and talked to a very nice young lady who was very well informed on this virus. She was great to talk to. I ordered your book, and I can't wait for it to get here so I can do some more learning. I haven't chosen an alternative way to go yet, but right now you're at the top of the list. I've got to get started soon to get on the reverse side of this virus before it starts getting the best of me.

I'm 46 years old and found out I've got hepatitis C in February. So, it's all new to me. I would still be in the dark if it wasn't for my computer, because the doctors don't tell you very much. I'm not too happy with them. It all started with me taking my 79-year-old mother to the doctor and then getting her meds at a pharmacy where they had a blood-pressure monitor. So while we were waiting, we checked ourselves out. Mom was fine. Mine was 180/120. My old momma freaked and started riding me to go to the doc, so I did.

My insurance has run out, so I went to the V.A. clinic; it was the first time I had gone there since I got out of the service in 1976. Well, the doc took all kinds of blood tests on January 17, and he calls me back about 2 weeks later and tells me I have hepatitis C virus. He told me I should quit drinking. He didn't tell me very much else. He set me up with a liver biopsy. Well, I got on the computer to find out more about this virus and I got pissed off. I wasn't sure what to think about our V.A. clinic or the doctors that work there, but their ethics suck!

So I went down there and bitched, but it didn't do much good. They just try to make you feel like something was solved and send you on your way, BS. Well, what was I supposed to do? A doctor calls you and tells you that you have a disease and it's very serious and don't spread it, and he didn't tell me much other than to quit drinking.

I don't understand why he didn't call me into his office and tell me and then have enough information to tell me about this hepatitis C, the do's and don'ts, etc. This still pisses me off!

After reading about your way of going on this, it sounds more helpful than interferon and all its side effects. I don't think I want to do it the way they suggest. I went to the gastroenterologist and they said that a hepatitis clinic would get in touch with me in probably 4 or 5 months, and I wouldn't be considered for interferon till that time. Also the gastro didn't have my liver biopsy results, so they got my paperwork all messed up. Jesus! So anyway, I'm waiting for your book, and I want to read it before I make a decision on what to do. Do you have any suggestions for me or wisdom? I'm open for anything and it is deeply appreciated.

Thanks for listening to me,<br>Rick

Dear Rick,

First let me say that 65% of veterans from the 60s and 70s have hep C. Many got it from a Gamma Globulin shot, which is something they gave as a hep B vaccine. Also the air gun, for giving shots. Regardless of how you got it, it is time to get rid of it. My program works better than anything currently offered. Try to stay away from the doctors except for blood tests.

I suggest that you avoid the liver biopsy, unless you want to know exactly what your condition is. They have to give you one before they give you interferon. I think interferon is poison and that it doesn't work.

I am here to answer any questions when you get through reading my book.

Thank you,<br>Lloyd

## Reached the End of Our Rope

Mr. Wright,

Ran across your web site while in search of something to help my husband. James was diagnosed with end-stage liver disease from hepatitis C and liver cirrhosis in April

2001. At the time, they told him he had a 50% chance of surviving 3 to 5 years without a transplant. By May, they had changed it to a 50% chance of surviving one year. There are no signs of cancer, thank God. His 48-year-old sister died of liver cancer caused by hepatitis C in March 2000. They never decided where she got it.

James is a 54-year-old Vietnam veteran and was going to the V.A. at the time of his diagnosis. We have owned and operated our own businesses for the past 20 years and we did not have health insurance at the time. The V.A. in Houston does not do liver transplants, and he was referred to Methodist Hospital.

We were told to get rid of all assets and close the business in order to apply for SSI and receive Medicaid to cover him for the liver disease, because the V.A. helps pay for heart and kidney transplants in Houston, but not liver!

We did as we were told and were forced to apply to the V.A. for assistance by the Social Security office. They awarded James a needs-basis pension of $715 per month. This made him ineligible for the SSI and much-needed Medicaid. It was too much money. His case for regular Social Security disability is still being reviewed. Even if he gets that, it takes two years for the Medicare to take effect after it starts. We tried to apply for just the Medicaid and were told to go to County Indigent Health Care. He is ineligible for that because he can go to the V.A. for medical treatment. But they don't do liver transplants in Houston!

The V.A. doctor said he could try to get on their list and have the transplant done in Pittsburgh. But that would require moving there and waiting for a liver, if he could be placed on their list. According to his V.A. doctor, his chances are very slim of getting on the V.A. list. And the time factor involved is too long.

Anyway, we were told to apply for the Texas High Risk Insurance and Methodist would do the evaluation and get him on the list. We did that, and he was approved for the insurance starting August 1, 2001. But they will not cover the liver for at least a year. So the doctor at Methodist said she will not do the evaluation (which, by the way, Methodist hospital will supply at no cost), because then she would have to put him on the transplant list, and they would be obligated to do the transplant even if it had not been a year since his insurance started.

So here we are four months later, and still nothing is being done. We have gotten rid of our only means of support. I cannot go outside and work because of James' condition, and nobody wants to do anything to help us get him medical treatment. Plus, $368 a month of the $715 he gets has to go to pay for the insurance. James became totally disabled in April 2001. He does not drink, smoke, or do drugs. He cannot take the interferon treatments because his platelet count stays at 40,000 or below. Last time they checked, it was 36,000. Seems from the point he started being so-called "treated" by the doctors with diuretics and such, he has gone downhill.

We have talked to, written, faxed, and emailed everyone we can think of and everyone else can think of trying to get some help. We have about reached the end of our rope. The doctors will not prescribe anything for his insomnia, nerves and restlessness. We have tried everything we can think of to try to alleviate it. If taking herbs will help, he will gladly try that. We just don't know what to take or how much. This condition has become so nerve-wracking that James has said he understands why some people commit suicide. I feel so helpless because I don't know what to do anymore. Any assistance you can offer will be greatly appreciated. I am enclosing a check to order your book in hopes of getting some valuable information to help us out.

Thank you,
Dawn

Dear Dawn,

When you read *Triumph Over Hepatitis C*, you will discover that I too experienced a very difficult time that appeared to be the end. Standing at death's door is very much different from contemplating it. I tried to get SSI disability and failed. I tried every option I could find and was denied. Life was bleak.

Several doctors had given me 3 to 5 years to live at best, and they suggested I get my papers in order and hope the medical community came up with some new treatment in time. I was not ready to die yet, and that is why I wrote *Triumph Over Hepatitis C* for people in your situation. If a carpenter like me could recover from a terminal condition, then so can you! With no money, but much will and persistence, I prevailed. I suggest that you have your husband take the following:

Milk thistle 400 mg 3 times per day
Lipoic acid 200 mg 3 times per day
Selenium 400 mcg per day
Dandelion root tea, 1 quart/day, afternoon and evening.

These few items can make a big difference. Dr. Berkson has a study that claims he takes people off the liver transplant list using the first 3 of these items. I can provide these items for you at cost.

In good health,
Lloyd

## Infected After Birth of Second Child

Dear Lloyd,

Thanks for your answer to my question about reishi vs. maitake mushrooms. I was infected in 1976 through an injection of RhoGam following the birth of my second child. I remember the acute infection, which resulted in the removal of my healthy gallbladder. I am currently asymptomatic and was diagnosed after I sustained a needle stick injury at work, where I am a licensed practical nurse. No one knows I'm sick unless I tell them. My liver enzymes are within normal limits and my viral count is below half a million. I have genotype 1a.

I was never interested in any "therapy" involving interferon injections. One look in the PDR convinced me that this was not the answer. With the abysmal success rate (an herbal would be laughed off the planet if it were this unsuccessful), and warnings concerning depression with suicidal ideation (to which I have been prone since childhood), the prospect scared me to death.

Then I joined some online hep C communities, and chatted with many, many people who had gone through the mono or the combo therapies, and had gotten to undetectable virus levels, only to have the virus come back with a vengeance. My plan was to wait. I knew I had time. A very close friend began doing research, and we've added supplements one at a time. I was thrilled to find your web site. Finding someone who has actually beaten hepatitis C by these means makes it so much easier to continue on, despite the expense. I do plan to buy your book, and your thymus extract looks like a winner, too. Thanks for putting the web site up and giving me hope!

Cathy

## Stayed in Bed Depressed for Two Years

Dear Lloyd,

I was diagnosed with HCV in October 2000; I've had it for 31 years. I have early cirrhosis. ALT 235, AST 187. Viral load one million; geno type 2b. My family wants me to take interferon and pegylated. I say no, so now a compromise: I try your stuff for 4 months, and if I don't see any good from it, then I go on interferon. To tell you the truth, I don't want to do interferon period.

I am soon to be 56 years old (grandma), and I'm in terrible shape. I stayed in bed depressed for 2 years and am now 125 lbs. overweight. Now I understand why I was so sick, tired, and depressed; it was the HCV. Now, I'm not so depressed and have been pretty normal, except when I catch something or am really tired.

Right now, I take 40 mgs. of Paxil for depression. I have been on it for 5 years, and every time I try to get off, my family begs me to get back on because I'm such a bitch. (Could you imagine me on the combo?)

I read your book and I believe you were cured. So, here are my questions: If I take everything you recommend, exactly how much money will your products cost me each month? There is a synthetic thymus medicine available in Mexico, I believe. It is called Zandaxian. It's probably the same stuff as from Singapore; it is also used in Italy, Africa and some other countries. What's your take on it?

Thank you,
Celeste


Dear Celeste,

Natcell Thymus is different from the chemical synthetic you mentioned, and works much better. In fact, there is no

113

comparison. The program is about $800 a month, plus shipping. You need to lose weight because that has a tremendous effect on liver function.

In good health,<br>Lloyd

## I Became the Epitome of Road Rage

Dear. Mr. Lloyd Wright,

I was diagnosed with hep C in August of 2000. I am 23 years old. When I was 18 months old in 1978-79, I was diagnosed with intussusception of the bowel. Some time in between there, I had lost a lot of blood.

I was taken care of at an army medical center. They gave me a blood transfusion, but my body rejected it. My dad told me I became beet red, and when I was stabilized, they sent me to Balboa Hospital.

Recently, I have tried the interferon treatment for only one month and I had to stop because I became the epitome of road rage.

I have read your book and believe what you say to be true. Please, I am so young. Can you help me? I would appreciate it very much.

Sincerely,<br>Deborah

Dear Deborah,

I suggest that people do exactly as I did, which is detailed in my book *Triumph Over Hepatitis C*.

The nature in which you caught this virus and the time factors can play a significant role in how your body deals with it. If you get started now, you can probably beat it before it gets you. It is kind of hard to explain, but when people get it at a very young age, usually their immune system deals with it in a somewhat different fashion than when people get it under the influence of drugs at an older age. You have a better chance.

Interferon does not work, and usually makes people sicker. Read *Triumph Over Hepatitis C.*

In good health,
Lloyd

## Why Would I Want to Inject Something Into My Body That Harms Me?

Dear Lloyd,

I know you can't make any promises, but I know your program could only do well for me, unlike the interferon. I started interferon because of a medical doctor, and stopped it because of common sense. Why would I want to inject something into my body that is only bringing harm to me, and I would only have a 10-20% success rate?

Mahalo from Hawaii,
Deborah

## It's the Little "One-On-Ones" That Help Me Right Now

Dear Lloyd,

I wanted to thank you for taking time from your schedule to talk with me twice now over the phone. I have ordered the thymus and adrenal as suggested, and I have been diligently taking everything else you suggested. I will say this, although I know it is early in my treatment, I don't seem to feel as tired or dragged out.

I have almost finished reading your book, and it's very easy reading. Thank you. I can relate too much of your life experiences and adventures prior to seeking a healthier alternative to living. The more I read and research, the more I am convinced that this was the right choice for me to make. I was thrilled to find your references to God in all this. Before coming to you, God has been a large part of my life over the last few years.

After nearly dying from a drug and alcohol consumed life, I woke up one morning, looked to the heavens, and cried out to the Lord, "Please don't let me die like this." My prayers were answered. After numerous attempts at trying things my way to no avail, I finally knew there was only one way, God's way and in his time. I have been clean for 11 years, have two beautiful daughters, a successful home-based business, and a relationship with God. I orchestrate praise and worship with the children at our church. I don't believe in coincidence, and I am even more sure of this after reading your story! You made a comment to me on the phone when I expressed my faith and that I was a strong believer in that God already had a plan in store: You said, "He sent you to me." I believe this to be true. I have no idea where this journey will lead, I don't really want to know all the details, but I feel blessed to have found you. I pray that you will stay close while I go through this. I pray that the roadblocks will be few and successes will be many. I pray that I will continue to keep God close at hand through all He has in store for me. It's the little one-on-ones that helps me right now. This gets scary sometimes.

Thank you again,
Cheryl

Dear Cheryl,

This is a really beautiful message. I thank you very much. I love it when I meet a real Christian. I do not tell many people this, but when I was crushed by the bulldozer (read Chapter 1 of my first book), I was delivered to men by a host of angels. When I saw them, I knew what they were and what they were doing. It was the most peaceful time I have ever spent on this earth. Most would consider me crazy for that statement.

For many years after my grandmother died, I did not feel that I was doing whatever it was I was called to do. I was sort of lost. I am now sure that helping people with hep C is my calling for now. It sure seems to be working for a lot of people who would otherwise be suffering. It is difficult to conceive that a carpenter could have the most popular web site under "Hepatitis C" on AOL (with no experience in marketing and sell as many books as I have) and have the remarkable sales record I have at Amazon.com and Barnes and Noble with no experience. GOD is behind this.

In good health,
Lloyd

## Liver Damage From Overdose; Age 20

Dear Lloyd,

At 18 years old, I found out I had hepatitis C after being hospitalized for an almost tragic suicide attempt. I had a lot of liver damage because of the overdose, and the doctor was watching my levels very closely. The day I was leaving, I read my levels for the last time and noticed that I had tested positive for hep C. The nurse was very upset I had noticed, and both she and the doctor were very quick to rush me out of the hospital.

After dealing with this for two years, my doctor has recommended the interferon and Ribavirin treatment. As a

117

very independent 20-year-old, this is a very scary thing to be faced with. I work full time and am my sole support. I am very fortunate, and I have a very understanding and caring boyfriend, but I am afraid that it won't be enough with this gruesome treatment. After telling my doctor about my serious background of depression, he kind of pleasantly ignored my fear to go on interferon, a drug known to cause depression in numbers of people.

Any advice/suggestions you have would be greatly appreciated. Thank you for your time.

Sincerely,
Sara

Dear Sara,

My best advice is to try and avoid interferon. I believe my program works better than anything else currently available. I know it is a little costly, but you can do a lot for yourself even using part of it. Some have reversed the virus just by using part of it. At 20, you may find it easier to do.

Interferon and depression can be a deadly combination. I have heard more horror stories than most anyone. I have approximately 30,000 clients, so I hear far more than the average doctor. I have met a few people who could work on interferon, but generally it is impossible. On my program, you will feel better than ever while you get well, something not yet heard of by the American medical machine.

In good health,
Lloyd

## They Made Us Practice Giving Injections, And the Needles Were Not Always Clean

Dear Lloyd,

I'm a 50-year-old heating and sheet-metal contractor. I tested positive for hep C about six months ago. I have never been sick from it, and I may have had it for 20 years or more. I'm still not sure how I got it, but I did do IV drugs a couple of times back in the mid-70s. Boy, would I like to turn that clock back! I was an assistant medic in my squad in Viet Nam; they made us practice giving each other field IV injections, and the needles were not always clean.

I had elevated liver enzymes in the mid-80s, and my doctor told me to stop drinking for six months, but I pretty much ignored him because I felt fine. I've been pretty much a happy-hour drinker (four to six pints of beer and a couple of shots a day) for the past 20 years. That's probably where a lot of my liver damage came from. No alcohol for six months now and I don't even miss it. This time when I had the high enzymes, the doc did a hep C test and it came back positive, 758,000 viral load, ALT 85, AST 74.

So the doctor sent me to the gastro man, and he sent me to get a biopsy and it showed fibrosis with portal bridging. He said that on a scale between 0 and 4 that I was a 2 1/2, and I should start the interferon injection torture immediately. I said, "screw you very much," and made a beeline to a homeopathic MD that was referred by a friend. He prescribed 10 autohem therapy sessions consisting of removing 200 cc of blood and running it through an ultraviolet light chamber to kill virus and then pumping it up with ozone gas and putting it back in. After every session, I felt greatly energized.

I discovered your web site and purchased your book, Hepastat, thymus, bulk licorice root, bulk reishi mushrooms and C ASPA SCORB. Your book is very inspiring, and I intend to add more of your herbal supplements to my regimen. After two months of the current protocol, my viral load is down from 758,000 to 575,000. I have every intention of beating this insidious, dark, and evil virus.

In the beginning, I had visions of having to go through with interferon injections and having to shut down my business, but with the natural course, I feel great and even more productive than before.

Yours truly,<br>Doug

## Rush to Give Blood Uncovers Disease

The following article was posted on Lloyd's web site on September 30, 2001:

### Hepatitis C Rates Higher Than Expected In First-Time Donors After Terrorist Attacks.

### By Carol Smith

Some of the first-time donors who rushed to give blood in the aftermath of the terrorist attacks are now discovering they may need medical assistance of their own in the future. More than twice as many people as expected tested positive for hepatitis C (a potentially debilitating liver disease) after donating blood, according to the records from the Puget Sound Blood Center.

"It's hard when someone finds out they have a disease such as hepatitis C," said Keith Warnack, spokesman for the Blood Center. "On the other hand, they found out something important that will help keep them healthy."

About 20 (0.7 percent) of the 2,712 first-time donors who turned out between September 11th and September 16th, tested positive for the disease even after disclosing no known risk factors. Their blood won't be used. "During typical blood drives, only about 0.3 percent of donors test positive for hepatitis C," Warnack said.

The data collected by blood banks around the country after the outpouring of donations gave public health officials a rare glimpse into the prevalence of the disease, which is believed to infect about two percent of the general population. Some health advocates, however, believe the rate could be much higher.

"Between 10 and 20 percent of people who test positive don't know how they contracted it," said Michael Ninburg, Executive Director of the Hepatitis Education Project, a Seattle-based group that provides support and information. Some risk factors include injecting drugs, having had a blood transfusion prior to 1992, or having received clotting agents before 1987. Having multiple sex partners also increases the risk.

"The health department has not seen the data yet," said Dr. Jeff Duchin, Chief of the Communicable Disease Control Program for Public Health, Seattle and King County. But the numbers did not surprise him. "The number of people reported to the Public Health Department has been growing as awareness has grown and more people have been tested," he said. "Some cases spontaneously resolve," he also said. But between 75 percent and 85 percent will develop into a chronic infection, and between 10 to 20 percent of those will eventually lead to cirrhosis of the liver.

Currently, hepatitis C is a leading cause of liver transplants in the country. "Avoiding alcohol is the primary method of reducing damage from hepatitis C," said Duchin.

# FOUR

# THE HYPOCRITICAL OATH

In a society motivated increasingly by greed, today's doctors seem to have forgotten the Hippocratic Oath, which has been taken for 2,000 years by physicians entering the practice of medicine. The oath was originally ascribed to the ancient Greek physician Hippocrates; that's how far back it goes.

Many contemporary medical schools use a revised and modernized version of the oath as an admonition and an affirmation to which their graduating classes assent. The current version approved by the American Medical Association is as follows:

> *You do solemnly swear, each by whatever he or she holds most sacred*
> *That you will be loyal to the Profession of Medicine and just and generous to its members,*
> *That you will lead your lives and practice your art in uprightness and honor,*
> *That into whatsoever house you shall enter, it shall be for the good of the sick to the utmost of your power, your holding yourselves far aloof from wrong, from corruption, from the tempting of others to vice,*
> *That you will exercise your art solely for the cure of your patients, and will give no drug, perform no operation, for a criminal purpose, even if solicited, far less suggest it,*

*That whatsoever you shall see or hear of the lives of men or women which is not fitting to be spoken, you will keep inviolably secret,*
*These things do you swear. Let each bow the head in sign of acquiescence.*
*And now, if you will be true to this, your oath, may prosperity and good repute be ever yours; the opposite, if you shall prove yourselves forsworn.*

The stories and letters in this chapter reflect the public's growing exasperation with our national healthcare system, to the point that we feel the "Hippocratic Oath" has become a hypocritical oath. The "modern" version of the Oath listed above still refers to doctors making house calls, yet many of my clients complain that physicians won't even return their phone calls in a reasonable amount of time, much less come to their home. In a humorous television commercial for a stock-brokerage firm that aired recently, a kindly old family doctor is seen making a house call on a young female patient he has attended for 30 years. Yet, how many of us even remember the time when doctors still made house calls in real life? Physicians haven't done that for decades. And the doctor in the commercial is also selling stocks during his house calls! Do you suppose this mythical doctor in the television advertisement is pushing stocks for the pharmaceutical companies?

It is my personal belief that many people would be alive today if they had learned of alternative methods of healthcare for hepatitis C earlier on in their treatment. As you can see from the first account listed below, I lost a respected friend to this illness. I only wish he could have benefited from my alternative healthcare solution sooner.

## If I Had Met Roy One Year Earlier,
## He Would Be Alive Today

A soft, gentle man will be greatly missed. Roy, my mailman, died June 5th, 2001, from the complications of hepatitis C. He was 46 years old. Roy's viral load was 200.000. His ALT 45, AST 79.

I first met Roy in December of 2000. One of the mail clerks at my post office asked me about the many packages I mail daily. I told her I am the author of a book called *Triumph Over Hepatitis C* and that sending out copies to numerous sufferers was keeping me quite busy. She immediately told me that one of her USPS peers was in a coma at a Kaiser hospital due to hepatitis C.

Knowing that the hospital, any hospital, was the worst place he could possibly be, I arranged to be introduced to him. I went to the hospital and saw Roy. He was given Natcell Thymus and Natcell Liver twice daily.

Soon Roy was back at work 12 hours a day delivering mail. However, it was clear that Roy's body was in a serious, irreversible state of decline.

Roy was so concerned about his health, he moved out of Malibu to be as close to the hospital as he could get. He wanted easy access, so that each time he required hospitalization he would be close.

After four comas and numerous procedures, it was clear that all the hospital could–or would–do was the minimum, and it appeared to me they were just waiting for Roy to die. Roy told me that he was on the transplant list and was awaiting a new liver. It was quite clear that a new liver would not have done Roy much good, if any.

My position was, and still is, that the best that could be done for Roy was to attempt to improve his quality of life for the time that he had left. Roy had gone through interferon treatment without success.

Roy had a buildup of lymphatic fluids in his abdomen and lower extremities that had to be mechanically removed several times. I wanted to help this man live out the rest of his life comfortably.

Initially, Roy consumed Natcell Thymus and Natcell Liver twice daily. He went through one case of aloe vera juice and one pound of dandelion root tea the first month. In December and January, he used three boxes of Natcell Thymus and five of Natcell Liver. He went back to work looking and feeling healthy. Then he stopped until March 20, when he purchased two boxes of Natcell Liver and one Natcell Thymus.

In the very beginning, Roy was yellow, his skin was pale, and he appeared very weak. After the first month on the program, his fellow postal workers began telling me that he really looked good. He was coming to work with enthusiasm, and he really did look much better. He said he felt much better and no doubt his liver was celebrating.

It seems one of the major problems with our medical community's current treatment of hepatitis C is this: Doctors do not tell their patients about the complications arising from hepatitis C. There are strict guidelines that dictate if a person is a viable candidate for a liver transplant. For example, if someone has additional life-threatening issues that a liver transplant will not remedy, well then, those people are ruled out.

Roy told me Kaiser had him on a liver transplant list, and he believed when the time came he would get one. Roy began having serious stomach infections after his last visit to the hospital. He no longer took the rejuvenating thymus and liver supplements, and he spent the last 28 days of his life in intensive care.

I sincerely believe if I had met Roy one year earlier he would be alive today. Roy was a soft gentle man. He will be missed greatly.

Lloyd

## Doc Callous and Lacking Compassion

Dear Mr. Wright,

I read your book tonight and appreciate your insight and courage. I particularly liked how there was no sanctimonious preaching, but just an honest conveyance of what worked for you and what you experienced.

I learned of my hepatitis C diagnosis in September when I went to doctor for "itching" symptoms, which, by the way, have not gone away. Went to a gastro, had a biopsy that showed "mild fibrosis," and was totally pissed off by the doctor's callous attitude and lack of compassion.

Because I am otherwise strong and healthy, he did not recommend interferon. As I am a 1-A type, he didn't think it would do any good. He told me to come back in three years for another biopsy. He told me I would have cirrhosis by the time I was 58. Also, he said he couldn't do anything else to help me. Thanks in advance for your help.

Patsy

## Sometimes Doctors are Blind

This individual in the next letter has had hepatitis C for over 30 years. He is in his mid 70's, and he is recovering quite well.

Dear Lloyd,

I went to my doctor for my 6-month checkup, and he told me there was no significant change in my condition. Do you agree with him? I've been on your treatment 6 months. Here are my test numbers:

| Date | AST | ALT |
|------|-----|-----|
| 05/17/2000 | 99 | 126 |
| 12/16/2000 | 63 | 70 |

Joe M.

Dear Joe

Try not to believe the doctor; he does not know. The people on interferon are confused and even lost.

There is a cure, and I see it happening. You can read about what happens to people on my message board. Some people take longer than others, but you are doing very well. I cannot believe your doctor can look at these test results and say you are not getting better. He must be blind!

Keep it up; you will see even more improvement.

Lloyd

## Variations on the Testing Theme-Phone conversation

Robert C. told me his doctor had called him and told him there had been no change since his last test. Upon further examination of the tests, I saw there actually was change.

Robert started on the program outlined in *Triumph Over Hepatitis C* on August 2, 2000. At that time his viral load was 2.5 million. On Dec. 21 it was less than 1 million. His ALT went up from 111 to 292, but he had pneumonia for a few weeks and was treated for it just prior to taking these tests. That could account for the rise in the ALT. I look forward to his next set of tests.

Lloyd

## After Confrontation, the Doc Agrees

Dear Lloyd,

I am writing to share my success and thank you for your work with the HCV. I am 48 years old. Although I did some wild and crazy things in the 70's, for the past 20 years I have maintained a lifestyle of healthy living.

This summer I applied for a life-insurance policy. Imagine my surprise and shock when I was denied coverage due to testing positive for the HCV.

I went to the Web and read stories of doom and gloom from the medical community. Then I visited your site! I ordered your book immediately.

In the meantime, I went to my family doctor who blew this off as "no big deal." He said it was like being on a slow moving train on a long track, and that I would probably live with it, rather than die from it. He said I should probably have a follow-up in about a year, and he gave me the name of a gastroenterologist.

Your book came and I read it the first night. I ordered the supplements right away and tried to follow your regimen as closely as possible, including the Natcell Thymus, which, as you know, is very expensive.

I went to the gastroenterologist, and he wanted me to start interferon. I said "No it's not really known to work." He agreed. He wanted to schedule me for a liver biopsy. I said, "No, it isn't really going to alter my course." He said, "Start taking milk thistle; it's the only known thing to work." He didn't say how much to take or where to get it. That was O.K. I already knew.

I had been on the supplements for about a week when I went to my chiropractor. He said to me, "I don't know what it is, but you're putting your body through some tremendous changes." That's when I told him about the HCV and starting the homeopathic supplements. He altered his technique that day to work on the area of the spine that controls the liver function.

I am happy to report that after only 5 weeks of your therapy in combination with my chiropractic treatments, my SGOT (AST) has decreased from 86 to 38 (a reduction of 56% that in some lab reference ranges is considered to be within the normal). My SGPT, (ALT) has decreased from 112 to 54 (a reduction of almost 52%). Viral load was not drawn on the first set of labs, so I have no baseline, but on the second lab draw my viral load was 8,000.

I recently added milk thistle and mushroom teas to my regimen. Again, thank you for sharing your work.

Sincerely,
Al

## Doc Tells Him Diet Doesn't Matter

Lloyd,

When your book arrived, I read it through. I can identify with your journey. I was diagnosed HCV in December 1997. I think I have had it for 20 years. I never really took anything until January 5th, 2000, when my AST was 126, my ALT was 294, and I was feeling terrible.

My naturopath/herbalist had me on the items listed below. I felt worse for three days then I started feeling better enough to go to this guy and praise him for helping

130

me. After a month, I just couldn't reach the next level of improvement. I was not really feeling that sense of well-being you write about in your book.

I am jazzed to announce that on July 6th, 2000 my AST was 68 and my ALT was down to 127. However, I was still not feeling very good. Now that I've started the Natcell Thymus, added the teas you suggested, and implemented a much more strict diet, I am certainly looking forward to my next test within the next couple weeks.

The gastroenterologist I just saw last week said that I should not take anything that would stimulate my immunity, and that I could eat anything I wanted. He said my diet didn't really matter. Some day soon these people will have to get the real message, don't you think?

Well, enough about me. Please continue to update the emails on your site. It sure gives me hope to know that others are getting well with this regimen.

Here are the items I began taking January 6th, 2000 (prior to Natcell Thymus): German Milk Thistle, Alpha Lipoic Acid, Homocystein Modifier, L-Methionine (Amino Acid), B-Complex, Lipotropic 1000, and Barlean's Flax Oil. I drink lemon water periodically throughout the day, followed with carrot, cucumber, and beet juice. And I eat plenty of raw vegetables.

Also, I'm certain to limit or eliminate the following: sugar, caffeine, alcohol, colas, dairy, fried foods, animal protein.

Thank you friend,<br>
Tom S.

## Doctor's Reaction Makes This Client
## Doubly Ready for Herbs

Dear Lloyd!

Went to a gastro doctor yesterday, and boy, he really took the wind out of my sails. He wants to put me on pegylated combo therapy for a 48-month trial. He was polite enough not to say it, but I got the feeling he thinks the herbal route is "B.S."

Anyway, I'm doubly ready to order. Could you tell me two things? One, do you know of any chat site that folks might be on? And two, since the thymus comes frozen, is it next-day delivery from the order date? I want to make sure I'm home when it gets here. Thanks so much for being there. I'd be really bummin' if it weren't for you.

Sammy

Dear Sammy,

I stay away from chat sites because someone is always online who has an entire following that believes interferon and their doctor is the only way. They blast me with thousands of snake-oil emails. I prefer to spend my time with reasonable people.

The thymus is frozen and is shipped overnight. If you make a note on the order which day you would like it delivered, I can accommodate that. Or you can call and tell me which day.

I enjoy putting results on my message board, and if you wish to put your email there, you could develop your own chat room.

Lloyd

## Doc is Just Going To Monitor Me

Lloyd,

I have come to realize that you are the only one that can help me with my problem. I plan on ordering products directly from you. I am still taking the products that you suggested and I feel great.

I need to get started with the thymus extract as soon as I can and maybe you can help me overcome this terrible virus that is in my blood and liver before it kills me. HaHaHa! It is not funny, but sometimes I think it is a dream and not real.

My doctor tells me I will live a normal life expectancy. What a lie! He says he can't do anything for me and he is just going to monitor me. So I will order some more products soon. You do have the best prices on all the products.

Thanks a lot for all the advice Lloyd, so far I feel pretty good.

Thanks!
Rodney

## Can't Find a Specialist for This Disease

I am a psychologist in California. I am presently treating an individual who has been drinking for many years and is newly clean and sober. She will be going to another specialist (MD) again. I use that term loosely, because I have found no specialists for this disease, forgive the cynicism.

She probably has toxic hepatitis plus a fatty liver from alcoholism. Will this alternative treatment increase or decrease the overall physiological effects of her addiction related problems?

Thanks for your input,<br>Dorothy, Ph.D.

## What a Bedside Manner!

Mr. Lloyd Wright,

I am a 53-year-old male with major liver problems complicated by a diagnosis from a blood test that I have hepatitis C. I am forced to use the Veterans Administration hospital and clinics for my tests and diagnosis. I am to go for a CAT scan and liver marker test in the next week. I am violently ill on a daily basis, and go back and forth between nausea, diarrhea, and constipation.

To date there has been no biopsy performed on my liver, only an ultrasound that indicated spots on my liver and severe cirrhosis.

My doctor has already told me that it doesn't look good for my future (what a bedside manner). When I mentioned milk thistle and other herbs as alternatives to their more invasive approach, he said herbal therapy is a waste of money and time. I have the desire to live a full life. Any encouragement from someone who's been there would be helpful. I am in the process of buying your book.

Thanks,<br>Gary

## Doctors Not Concerned About My HCV

Dear Lloyd,

I found your web site this week and have decided to order your book. I too am disheartened by the medical care that is available for hep C and the doctor's lack of knowledge and care.

I was first diagnosed in 1995 when I was preparing for an upcoming hip-replacement surgery. They tested my blood and informed my surgeon. He told me it must be an old infection and he was not concerned. However, I was alarmed by it and went to my MD and was retested. The diagnosis was confirmed. My MD told me that there is no cure, but it could be treated when it becomes a problem.

As time passed and the medical industry forced us into HMOs, I could no longer see those doctors and be covered by my insurance. In 1998, I selected my HMO primary-care doctor and entered on the forms that I had hep C. The doctor reviewed my forms, and he did not even bring it up when he talked to me.

When I was feeling bad and seeing him concerning my lack of energy and dizziness, he proceeded to run heart tests and other blood tests. After all the testing, he informed me he couldn't find anything wrong.

In 1999, I decided to change primary-care doctors and went to see a second physician with the same complaints. They also ran a series of tests to check for low-blood sugar, blood clots, and respiratory problems and found nothing they could target in on. They still did not seem to be concerned about my hep C problem.

So I took to the Internet to do research on my own, only to find myself looking death in the face and with very little hope. After previewing your site, I find that there may be a light in the far distance in this tunnel of despair.

I noticed on the message board that you were using test results to gauge the progress. This leads me into the following questions you may be able to answer for me:

What type of doctor do you recommend I seek out as a specialist to follow my hep C? What type of tests should I request and what are the things I should look for? How long will it take following your program to see if I can be cured? How much will the cost be associated with following your recommendations?

Thanks,<br>Murray

Dear Murray,

I suggest that you get a doctor who will give you blood tests once every three months, a liver panel, and a HCV PCR viral load. Other than that, forget about doctors unless you have some sort of emergency.

Fax or mail me the blood work you have. Read my book, and use my program as much as you can afford. After three months, you will have a smile on your face. In a few weeks, you should feel better. Some people take a little longer, some a little less.

It costs about $700 to $1,100 dollars a month, depending on how much of the program you do. Some people choose to use the Natcell Liver as well as the thymus, and that costs an additional $285 extra a month. Those people who use the liver as well as the thymus have a quicker response.

You need to have an iron-binding test. Males often have an iron overload in their liver, and it is easy to remedy. A few phlebotomies usually will take care of it. If you have an iron overload, it takes longer to get well unless you do the phlebotomies.

It took me 18 months to get hepatitis C free. I have had some people clear the virus in a shorter time. Many do the program for a while then feel better and stop, thinking they are fine. Plus, they need to use the money for other things. Some come back later and start over.

Hepatitis C does not go away overnight. Americans are conditioned to take a pill for a week or two and then think their health problem is over. Combating hepatitis C takes a lot of effort and persistence. I hope that answers your questions.

Lloyd

## Docs Protect Their Zillion-Dollar "Good Thing" at the Expense of Our Lives

Dear Lloyd!

Don't let these MD a-holes get you down. They're protecting their zillion dollar "good thing" at the expense of our lives. I work with a lot of them and on the whole most of them are mindless wonders with their self-esteem boosted up by years of overpay, graft from drug companies bribing them successfully to dispense their products, and the AMA boosting their "credibility" and encouraging them to focus more on their own egos than on actual healing and curing.

I personally appreciate all you've done. The combination of herbs with no side effects has eliminated night sweats and side pains. I'm scheduling a PCR test that can only be ordered through an expensive specialist, probably a biopsy, and then I'll decide about live thymus.

Again, the work you're doing is so very important.

Thanks again,<br>Stephan

## Just Making Donation To Doctor's Retirement Fund

Hey, Lloyd,

I just finished reading your book. Excellent!

I will be shopping for some of your products. The thymus I found is in liquid form, and you use an eyedropper to put it under your tongue. It is called Thymus Support and is made by Natra-Bio. A lot of the things you suggest I have already been doing. Some of them are new to me.

I, like you, feel that when I go to the doctor I am just making a donation to his retirement fund. He is not doing anything, and it seems like he wants to wait till I take a turn for the worse before he acts. I went the interferon route along with Ribavirin. Enzymes went up as soon as I quit.

Since I took matters into my own hands, my energy level has skyrocketed and I need a lot less rest. I always waking up early, primed, and ready to go.

Thanks for the hope,

Betty


## Seems Like Doc Waiting for Him to Die

Dear Mr. Wright,

I just happened upon your web site while surfing the net looking for information on hepatitis C. My husband was diagnosed in August of 1999 with hepatitis C, and began a long, frightening and exhausting ordeal.

The arrogance of the medical community is mind-numbing. We have gotten to the point of such frustration with the doctors, who are supposed to be there to help, that my husband is now looking for new ones. Their arrogant, uncaring attitude has destroyed our faith.

He was supposed to start his interferon/Ribavirin treatment two weeks ago, but the doctor just pushed him aside, putting him off the day we had an appointment at the hospital for his first injection. Since then, we have not been able to get hold of the doctor, get a return call, or anything. It makes you feel like a non-person, a problem to be ignored or swept aside. My husband said he feels like they are waiting for him to slowly die. How sad to say about people who take an oath to help people.

I would very much like to hear from you; just a supportive word would be appreciated. I will be looking for more info on your site. Thank you for taking the time to read this.

Yours truly,
Pauline

## Docs Rank With Cops, Politicians, Lawyers

Dear Lloyd,

As usual, you have my permission to post anything I write to you on your message board. I don't care if you use my name or not. I am not ashamed of my disease; I'm PISSED. The people on interferon obviously don't know what the garbage is doing to their bodies and minds. I am scared to death of that stuff. I would rather stick to the program you suggest, feel good, and try to forget the prognosis offered by the hepatologist.

It's weird, when I left his office over a year ago with my ALF magazine, I felt really sick. But, I didn't feel sick the day before. Odd isn't it, that once a "doctor" says something you start to feel all the "symptoms." I walked out of there waiting for my fingers to club and ready to spit up blood. My right side hurt, and I was tired, weak, and ready to die. Every ten minutes I was looking in the mirror waiting for these bruises to show up, the ones that he was surprised I didn't have yet, when just the night before I was partying with the best of them.

Odd, how one authority figure can piss on your parade and blow your mind. Granted, I did my day at Woodstock a long time ago and really have been anti-establishment for 30 years or so, but I always respected doctors; they made you feel better. Now they are right up there with cops, politicians and lawyers, in my book.

I wish all heppers would rethink what poison they are putting in their system, and try something more natural like your program. Hey, if it doesn't work, they can always go back to the interferon; they can have my prescription!

As ever,
Vince

## Hurt By The Lack Of Communication

Dear Lloyd,

Again thank you for your help. At first, I was skeptical of new alternatives, but you so far seem to have the best handle on the hepatitis C virus. It's a good feeling to know that I am doing something to fight this dragon! We are lucky to have you share your knowledge with us.

This all started with a checkup last June. I had my biopsy two months ago, and have yet to have a hepatologist see or talk to me. I have not been told anything about what to eat and not drink. It scares me to think of all the people in my boat that are being hurt by this lack of communication. Well, you know all this.

Thanks again,
David

## Docs Thought of as Royalty

Dear Lloyd,

Got your book. Read it in two days, and now I'm re-reading it again. Very helpful and informative and enjoyed it. Sorry you had to go through so much shit to get here, but I guess it's a blessing for you and the rest of us. By the way, you can put the last letter I wrote on your web site.

I'm starting to have contempt for the MD's that I see at the V.A. Ten years of study, and they learn that if they can't dazzle 'em with brilliance, they will baffle them with bullshit!  Or they pass the buck to somebody else! I'm starting to think that the doctors that they hire at the V.A. are not the cream of the crop, but exactly the opposite. In fact, most of them are from other countries and don't speak and understand our language very well. Or, the protocol in their country was different. Are all doctors thought of as being like royalty?

I asked this Irish doc yesterday what he thought about chiropractors. It ruffled his feathers and he boasted about how much education he had and that he taught for ten years. I heard more about that than what I went in there for. And you know, to tell you the truth, I have no idea why they wanted me to see this guy. There was nothing done in that office except BS.

Rick

## Doc Made a Face and Smirked

Dear Lloyd,

My husband heard about you on the radio, and we ordered your book.  I read the whole thing today when I should have been working.

I even read part of it while I was waiting for an appointment with a gastroenterologist. I showed the book to her and asked if she had read it. She made a face and kind of smirked, and said no. I told her that I had already tried interferon and was not willing to do that again, and asked her if she could suggest a naturopathic doctor. She informed me that "Group Health" does not have such a program. I kind of figured that.

Your book is very helpful. Thank you. On page 199, I was stunned at the symptoms of this 40-year-old female. That is exactly what I have been complaining about for years. I even went to the doctor recently due to a MAJOR rash. She said there was no relationship between my rash and hep C.

Thanks again, and I am so happy that you have had such amazing results. What determination you have.

Arlene

## Can't Get Through to Docs

Dear Lloyd,

My name is Ralph, and I live in New Jersey. I'm 53 years old. I'm diagnosed with hep C. Over 3 years ago, I tried interferon for 6 months with no results.

I have your book. I hear you say a lot about getting government aid such as SSI Medicaid. I wouldn't worry about getting that. It does not help. It even hurts. The doctors do nothing for you. When you are a Medicaid patient, you're sent to clinics where you see different doctors every time you go who know nothing about your case or hep C.

I am not being treated with anything at the present. Been trying to get into a hep C clinic that they have at one of the hospitals in New Jersey; been waiting over 6 months and still no answer. If I had insurance, it would have taken me already.

I will not go on interferon any more. Your book sounds good. I go through the same things with doctors. I fight with them all the time, and hospitals; I can't get through to them. I feel very bad all the time. I would like to try your program. I would like to know how you were able to do what you did feeling this sick?

Thank you,<br>
Ralph

Dear Ralph,

My neighbors called me the "Ever Ready Bunny." I sold everything I owned, put things in the recycler that I did not think anyone would want, and parted with things that were dear to me, items owned by my grandfather and grandmother. I even hocked my grandmother's wedding ring. I did eventually get it back, as a friend of mine loaned me money and I used it for collateral.

Having been a carpenter for 30 years, I had worked for everyone in my neighborhood. I sold myself to them and some had compassion because of my condition and they tolerated my slower than normal performance.

You asked me how I did it? My answer is God did it!

In good health,<br>
Lloyd

## Hep C Just Floating in My Blood Stream

Dear Mr. Wright,

Thanks for trusting me enough to send me a copy of your book! I was shocked and elated to find it in my mailbox. I thank God for you and I am posting you a check immediately.

Since 1994, I have gone through some of the things that you experienced, and with the help of your book, I hope that I will not have to experience all of it.

I think my doctor just doesn't give a damn whether I live or die. She asked me the ages of my two kids and said that she'll have to make sure that I will be around to raise them. I don't know if I'm depressed or not, since everything I say anything, someone wants to push a Paxil down my throat.

My hep doc doesn't see a need to treat me with anything. She says, "Interferon doesn't help anyway." I think it's mainly due to the fact that I am a Medicaid recipient.

My husband was a vet and died with hepatitis C. That was the only reason they tested me when I asked for the test. I was assured that it was not transmitted from him and the kids turned out negative.

I've been diagnosed with having a slew of ailments, and I received numerous prescriptions that I promptly trashed. The hep doctor says that if someone has to have hep C, I've got the unique one. It has run its course and hasn't done any liver damage or any other damage and its just floating along in my blood stream, I guess waiting for me to do something to suppress my immune system.

I know that I have presumed on your kindness in writing you a book, but you're the only person that I've met that I can talk to. If there is any way to buy your regimen, I will! I have to! I don't want to die just yet.

Received the book today, finished reading it 2 hours later. Thanks a million, Mr. Wright! I am telling everyone I know about you.

I remain forever in your debt and I'm grateful that God led me to you. I pray for your continued remission.

Sincerely yours,
Ceila

## Docs Full of What Comes Out of the South End of a Northbound Bull

Dear Lloyd,

I am 43 years old. I ordered, received, and have read your book. I was diagnosed with hepatitis C in June of 1999 after donating blood. The blood bank notified me. I saw my doctor, had confirming second-opinion testing, and he basically told me no symptoms, no worries. I immediately quit drinking, and have had no symptoms that I am aware of. I basically feel good.

I found out that when asked about hepatitis C, doctors are basically full of what comes out of the south end of a northbound bull. I read enough about interferon before reading your book to convince me that it is not for me and hopefully never will be.

I want to ask your opinion as to what combinations and dosages of your remedies might I be suited for. I am worried about overkill. Is that stupid or what? Thanks for your book and your help.

Robert

## I Guess No One Too Important Has Died of This Disease Yet

Dear Lloyd,

I have many questions to ask you and would like to talk to you about how society regards alternative medicine. For

145

God's sake, if you were able to triumph over this disease with herbs, then why isn't the medical field recognizing this?

My husband has a doctor's appointment with the University of Pennsylvania in Philly on August 31, and I will be talking to this doctor about you and give her the materials that I have found, along with your book, because I'm sure I will have your book read within 1 or 2 days. One of my questions to the doctor will be how she feels about alternative medicine, and if her response is negative, the second question I'm going to ask her is if she has ever tried it with any of her patients. If the answer is no, then I anticipate that the rest of the meeting is not going to go too well, and we'll be looking for another doctor.

I am very angry about our society. I guess no one too important has died of this disease yet. This is so widespread and is worse than having AIDS. I wish my husband had contracted that instead. It seems people with AIDS survive a hell of a lot longer. If your remedy really works, then why doesn't the health profession work with you?

I am thinking of taking a second job as a bartender to raise the money for my husband's treatment with your remedy, or somehow have a benefit to support him through the community. My work is cut out for me. If, after reading your book and doing some investigating, I'm happy with the results, count on my getting a six-month supply for my husband.

Thank you and I will be talking to you soon.

Kimberly

## Doc's Advice: Cheaper to Die From Hep C Than to Cure it

Lloyd,

Thank you very much for the book. I am going to use a translator later this week, and I'll let you know how it worked. I already started reading the book myself; it's very interesting. I can't wait to read the whole thing.

The book is for my brother-in-law, who was diagnosed with hepatitis C. He donated blood 2 years ago. About 2 weeks ago, he received a phone call from some institution telling him that they had found hepatitis C in the blood he donated 2 years ago! These people waited 2 years to inform him!

He just visited a doctor for advice. This doctor graciously told him that it was cheaper to die from hepatitis C than to cure it. This really upsets me.

I am a big fan of alternative medicine. I also use herbs for every single disease that bothers me from time to time. I am very disappointed of modern medicine. Thanks to a great doctor, who prescribed me herbs a long time ago as the treatment to follow, the horrible seizures that affected me for years disappeared forever. With just a 3-month treatment, my life changed for good, and the seizures never came back.

Before I found this doctor, I had visited who knows how many different clinics and specialists, who I'm sure had no clue about what they were doing or looking for. They just were not helpful. The only thing I noticed was that things were going from bad to worse. Well, I think you know the story.

Thanks again,
Sandra

### Where Are the Marcus Welby Types?

Lloyd,

Having been an R.N. and seen the inside of our physicians' "Godlike" personalities, I am saddened by any patient's non-responsive attitude toward an alternative treatment that would help them, regardless of how mad their doctor may get about it. In other words, ALWAYS QUESTION your doctors!

As I used to stand by watching a physician talk to family members, I would observe them cowering down into submission whenever they questioned something or asked about other alternative treatments. The almighty doctor would act as if someone put a stake in his heart, and how dare anyone question his treatment, because he is a specialist and should be treated with respect.

I've worked with cardiac units, respiratory, surgery, medical, and O.R. The doctors would not even attempt to see any altered course of any treatment, once THEY had made up their minds, and we (the nurses) would have to deal with the families and patients after the doctor left.

What has happened to the "Marcus Welby" types—doctors with caring, open minds, whose only concern curing and easing a patient's pain?

Even now, being a hep C'er, my doctor comes into the exam room, very stiff and sharp with me, always asking, "Hello, Susan, how are we now, are we still entertaining the quack's treatment?"

I usually tell him, "I am just here for blood levels to be drawn, and no, no quackery, just sound natural medicine. And you still can't explain why my levels are all now within normal limits, along with my blood pressure, since I got off your treatment."

So all we can do, Lloyd, is hope one day, the "Marcus Welbys" of this world will return.

Sue

Dear Sue,

I have not heard from you for a while. Hope you are still taking care of you and yours.

I love your messages; they reflect the real world.

Keep getting well.
Lloyd

Dear Lloyd,

I am doing good. That advice from you on MSM, wow, it took almost every ache away from my joints, so I am looking forward to what this aloe does. Heck, I even have my hubby on milk thistle, dandelion, and his regular vitamins. He's off caffeine and doesn't even know it. I buy him decaf and dump it into the red Folgers's can.

I decided since I am going to live a lot longer, I better have my honey around and healthy, too. I bake my own bread now too, and have become a connoisseur of the teas. I mix the reishi with the milk thistle and Celestial's lemon zinger, and it goes down way easier.

About a month ago, I noticed I don't have to sleep up on two pillows anymore; no more acid reflux at night, and I sleep thru the night. I mean, because of you, within a year I have gotten rid of EVERY symptom, and that's the plain truth.

Yes, it took a year, and some discipline and a gradual change in diet, getting rid of the bad foods we get in the habit of thinking we need, but a year ain't nothing.

You are definitely in our lives, daily. You stay healthy, you hear me!

Good, and keep up the great radio shows.

As always,
The Imp, Sue

Dear Sue

I just love reading your email. They are the ones that crack a smile on my face when I am going nuts from the stress of all the damage control from FedEx and shippers and stuff that goes wrong all day.

Keep getting well.
Lloyd

## Doc is Encouraging

Thank you, Lloyd Wright,

We appreciate your help. Jackie is doing really well. His family doctor has said to keep doing whatever it is we are doing. His last blood work came back perfect. Now, that was only regular blood work, not hepatitis counts. But we were really encouraged. His blood pressure is normal also.

I wish the medical community would look more into this treatment. Jackie is planning on going in September for more blood work specifically for the hepatitis. Thank you again for your great help. I feel like you and Katie are saving his life.

Karen

## Docs All Think Herbs Have Evil Things in Them

Dear Lloyd,

I respect your efforts, and I can believe the craziness that you're talking about! What you are doing requires someone who is staying on track, and more than motivated. I thank you for that!

I just want to tell you about the QUICK appointment that my husband and I had. We brought in your book, asked questions about the milk thistle and Hepastat. The doctor was not putting these things down. In fact, he thanked us for talking to him first. He said he has been very much interested in the "herbal" world, ever since his college days. But he is concerned about what is in the herbal tablets.

I can understand your feelings about the medical field and, oh my God, I do believe that they are corrupt, too, with the medicine they prescribe. But I just don't understand why they won't get this news out! Does it all come down to the ALMIGHTY BUCK?

People are dying! Even though the FDA has not approved of these herbs, can't they just tell people about them off the record? Or is it because of the lawsuits that could happen? I truly want to know WHY?

Thank you Lloyd!<br>Mary

Dear Mary,

I would forget about your doctor. They all think that herbs have evil things in them. No doubt some herbs do. I deal with very reputable companies that pride themselves on making the finest products.

The best way I can think to explain this thing between doctors and herbs is similar to the 1960s when, in the South, blacks rode in the back of the bus and used separate restrooms.

In the chapter of my book on albumin, there is a true story about doctors learning to wash their hands. Read it. It may give you some insight into how arrogant these people are.

Lloyd

## Begging for Help

Dear Lloyd,

I know you all probably get stuff from people begging you all the time. Well, I'm one of those beggars.

My husband will be #1 on the liver transplant list IF we can raise enough money. His doctor says he has only a few, probably two, months left. I am asking, no begging, for you to send this message on to others. Thanks,

His begging wife,<br>Beth

Dear Beth,

I have changed the lives of a few people who were in the state you describe. 1 or 2 vials of Natcell Liver a day and 1 vial of Natcell Thymus a day for at least 3 months.

My other suggestion is, and this is very serious and real, in Columbia they do liver transplants just as are done here in the United States, for $3,000. There is no waiting. Again, they have the same technology we have and are just as good. For an additional $2,000, you can arrange for in-home care for one month, as one needs to stay for a month near the hospital for treatment. I know this sounds hard to believe because we are all brainwashed by American rip-off artists.

In good health,<br>Lloyd

## America Owned and Operated By
## the Big Drug Companies

Greetings,

My fiancée has hep C, and I was wondering if there is a doctor in Los Angeles who takes our insurance and prescribes Natcell Thymus. We have started taking some of the supplements mentioned in the book. My fiancée also feels that she may have hypothyroidism. While reading the thyroid book, they mention T-cells and some of the stuff you talk about. I was wondering if Natcell Thymus would have any effect on the production of the T3 and T4 cells?

Sam

Dear Sam,

Many people with hep C have thyroid problems. Shortly after taking Natcell Thymus, the problem goes away. Some insurance companies do cover Natcell Thymus.

Lloyd

## Doctors Treat People Like Idiots, And
## Hate Jerks Like Me Who Ask Too Many Questions

Hello again,

Wow. It sounds like you were definitely dealing with doctors from the dark ages. It's really amazing that you went to hepatologists who didn't even mention virus genotype. But of course, so many doctors treat people like idiots. Their attitude towards them is that patients wouldn't understand their language anyway, which a lot of people don't. So many people blindly trust their doctors and don't ask questions.

I work as a medical transcriptionist for a hospital, but I've also been in nursing school and completed my bachelor's degree in medical records, so I was in the same anatomy and physiology, nutrition, epidemiology classes, etc, as the people who work in the front line of care–you know, "the real important people." It amazes me though, when I'm typing a history and physical on a person who has had multiple surgeries (which they cannot identify to the doctor), why the surgeries were performed. It is very common. Doctors hate jerks like me who ask too many questions, though, and just want me to get the heck out of their office once they're done examining me.

Anyway, the HCV virus genotyping test was one of the first things they identified me with as being positive for HCV. Thanks for writing back. God bless you for sharing your information with others, because I truly believe that pharmaceutical drugs are nothing but dangerous, and everything that goes into the body will have an effect somewhere. Our world is in such a mess, but it still doesn't stop people from reproducing. I think the religious fanatics figure the Lord will step in and fix what we've all screwed up and the greedy developers don't care. Greed and stupidity control the world, unfortunately.

Thanks again,<br>Rolf

Dear Rolf,

Please keep in mind that every day I speak with people from all walks of life, all across the country, who have been diagnosed with hep C, been through the interferon treatment, and do not have a clue what a genotype is. When I ask them, they ask their doctor, and they report back to me all sorts of different things that their doctor says.

Usually a genotype test was not performed. This is a common problem even today.

Lloyd

## Contracted Both Hepatitis B and C

Dear Lloyd,

I contracted both hepatitis B and C. I was wondering what chance of living and/or getting rid of them I have. I've talked to a couple of doctors, but they seemed to play me off and tell me I can go 25 years before it affects me. The University of Illinois is helping people with one or the other, but don't want to take me because I have both; that scares me. I was wondering if I can get some honest answer from you, Lloyd. Please help.

Thank you,<br>Paul

Dear Paul,

It may be that the university wants to study something different. It is true that B and C, if they are both active, do not respond well to interferon. My program will work on both B and C. People with just B get rid of it in a short time. The two together will be a little longer process. It can work, and the only problem is that it will be a little costly.

If I were you, I would be doing the alternative program. That is as honest as I can get.

In good health,<br>Lloyd

The following are excerpts from an ABC news program called ON THE MONEY TRAIL that aired on November 18, 2001 concerning a federal investigation into an alleged "payola" scheme between one Drug Company and doctors, for the sake of profits. These excerpts are posted on my web site message board.

## CHARLES GIBSON, ABC NEWS:

On THE MONEY TRAIL tonight, we look at how and why doctors choose specific drugs for their patients. An overwhelming majority of doctors simply choose the drug they think will work best. But the U.S. Attorney in Boston is investigating a case in which it is alleged one drug company helped doctors make huge profits if those doctors would prescribe the company's drug. Here's ABC's chief investigative correspondent, Brian Ross.

## BRIAN ROSS, ABC NEWS:

This Lewiston, Maine, urologist is one of four doctors indicted in a sweeping federal investigation of how a major pharmaceutical company allegedly offered big money to get doctors to prescribe a cancer drug called Lupron. Can we talk to you just for a second about....

## DR. JOEL OLSTEIN:

Well, I really don't think so.

## BRIAN ROSS, ABC NEWS:

According to the indictment, Dr. Joel Olstein, who says he is cooperating with authorities, made tens of thousands of dollars by taking free samples from drug company representatives and then billing insurance companies and Medicare for the full price. And according to authorities, it was all part of a campaign by the makers of Lupron to get doctors to prescribe the effective, but costly, prostate-cancer drug instead of its less expensive competitor.

## DR. GERALD WEISBERG:

It's bothersome to the extent that therapeutic decisions could be influenced by personal financial gain.

## BRIAN ROSS, ABC NEWS:

The scheme was presented to thousands of doctors across the country, according to Dr. Gerald Weisberg. He's the former head of clinical research for Lupron at the TAP Pharmaceutical Company in suburban Chicago, and has told federal authorities that the company concluded that many doctors cared as much about profit as they did about how good the drug was.

## DR. GERALD WEISBERG:

It was a pitch made on financial gain for physicians.

## BRIAN ROSS, ABC NEWS:

And that was widespread?

## DR. GERALD WEISBERG:

We are talking about schemes clearly implemented through the efforts of persons in the TAP home office and then given to the people out in the field.

## BRIAN ROSS, ABC NEWS:

Company officials say Dr. Weisberg is a disgruntled employee who was fired. But internal company documents obtained by ABC News reveal the kind of pitch the company made to doctors, including something called the Lupron Checkbook. It was designed to show doctors how they could make huge profits by purchasing Lupron at substantial discounts and billing health insurers for them at the full price, a secret arrangement the patients were never intended to know.

## DR. ARNOLD RELMAN, HARVARD MEDICAL SCHOOL:

And what it says is, "Doctor, how much do I have to give you in order to persuade you that my drug or my treatment is better than the other fellow's drug, or better than no drug at all?"

## BRIAN ROSS, ABC NEWS:

The Lupron investigation is a case that has closely been watched, and it may reveal a great deal about how big drug-company tactics can drive up prices and influence medical judgments. Brian Ross, ABC News, New York.

# *FIVE*

## CONVENTIONAL MEDICINE
## CAN KILL YOU

Conventional medical treatment is the third leading cause of death. The following messages reflect but a fraction of the "doctor stories" I hear every day. They are anguished, frustration-filled accounts of attempts by patients to deal with our conventional health care system and inability of that system to offer useful, high-quality information to those with hepatitis. I include this correspondence in a separate category to help you see that you are not alone in your search for understanding, information, and direction. "Physician error" is officially listed as the sixth leading cause of death. Unofficially, some tallies claim it is number one. In the first letter below, written by a chiropractor, he states that "conventional medicine" is the third leading cause of death. I think the statistics tell their own story, but I'll let you read about my clients' experiences for yourself. You be the judge.

### Tunnel Vision of the AMA/FDA

Dear Lloyd,

I received your book, and found it quite comforting and informative as well as entertaining. I can tell you that you were holding back concerning the arrogance and tunnel vision of AMA/FDA practices. My brother (tackling cancer slowly, but surely) has opened my eyes to the shortsightedness of conventional medicine. What a relief it was to hear that I might not have to expect a long, drawn-out death from HCV!

Thank you, Lloyd!<br>
Dale

## FDA Guinea Pig

Dear Mr. Wright,

I just got your book today. I am so glad I ordered it. I have had hepatitis C since 1988. Back then they didn't have a name for it. I was young and more or less forgot about it after I felt better. It came back to haunt me later. I was on Intron-A for three months the first time, off for three months, then on for six months. Each time my liver counts were going down for a while, then back up before the treatment ended.

After a year I became an F.D.A. guinea pig for the Intron/Ribavirin study for 48 weeks. I have never been so sick in my life. I did have a three-year remission. Now that it has returned, I have been worrying that I would have to return to the treatment that cost me 11 months of my life, my job, and my health. The cure nearly killed me. Then I found you on the net. I am so excited I can hardly wait.

Thank you,<br>
Jacob B."

Dear Jacob,

I would love to put your email on my message board. It is very informative. The program I outline in *Triumph Over Hepatitis C* works and you will feel good while doing it.

Lloyd

Dear Lloyd,

Yes, please use any of my messages on your message board. Maybe it will help someone else to get started in the right direction. The cure doesn't have to be worse than the illness.

We are very grateful to have found you on the net. THANK GOD I don't have to be made sicker to feel better by so called modern medicine.

Jacob B.

## Releasing the Stigma

Dear Lloyd,

It wasn't until I said I had hepatitis C that people started coming out of the woodwork. There is an awful stigma attached to this out here. I don't care who knows. I even let the staunch doctor at the hospital know exactly where I think I got this "gift": right at his hospital after a transfusion 19 years ago after my son's birth. Of course you know many other explanations came flowing from his mouth. But the bottom line is that it doesn't matter where any of us got it, it's how we are going to cure it.

Take care. As ever,
Valerie

## Doctor in Denial, Calls Case "Spontaneous Remission"

Dear Lloyd,

I have hepatitis C and have been through all the conventional treatments of interferon. I initially had 6 months of injections of 3 million units 3 times per week. But my counts still weren't normal.

Then, my doctor referred me to the University of Florida, Shands Teaching Hospital, where Dr. Gary Davis was conducting a study for Schering-Plough. The study used the same treatment of 3 million units 3 times per week. When I still had high AST ALT levels, I was then given 5 million units 3 times week. I developed such horrendous side effects my doctor contacted Dr. Davis and had me removed from the study. When I stopped the study my AST was 128 and my ALT was 189. That was after several years of the interferon combination treatment.

During the course of this extended treatment, I got mouth sores, lost most of my hair, and was constantly exhausted and sick to my stomach. I also saw things that were not there, and I became increasingly depressed. In my case, I had never experienced depression in my life and I am in my 50s. I now live with depression.

I had been told that interferon would leave your body once you stopped taking it. But in my case, there seems to have been permanent damage to my brain pathways. It also affected my memory and I now have ADD.

Since my liver is already in advanced cirrhosis, I started taking milk thistle tablets as well as other parts of your program against my doctor's advice. My ALT is now 32 and my AST 35. Of course my doctor still isn't convinced, and he won't be until it's proven by medical science that your program, instead of a *spontaneous remission*, healed me."

Steve H.

**Would Rather See A Vet Than An MD**

This 37-year-old pharmacist started my program in February 2000 after trying six months of the combo

162

therapy. His wife called me, saying her husband was losing weight and his skin was a pale gray color. He was consistently fatigued, unable to work a full day, and his personality was fading.

After just two weeks on my program, another call from his wife confirmed that the color had returned to his skin and that he was feeling and acting healthier.

Thirty days later, she reported that he had begun to gain weight, and that his personality was back to the way he was when they were first married.

He currently no longer feels sick. However, his blood tests indicated only a slight drop in his numbers. But this information is reported from his doctor; the client never saw his tests.

This client continues on the program with great expectations. He stated that he would "rather see a veterinarian for hepatitis C than a doctor."

Lloyd

## Doc Says, "Time To Re-educate Myself"

One of my clients, who had purchased my book, called me. He had started using the remedy outlined in my book.

This man has known his doctor since his doctor was a child. Five years ago, his doctor told him that he had cirrhosis and hepatitis C, and the only way to treat it was with interferon. The man refused, and he kept getting sicker. Then he ran across my web site back in January, gave me a call, and went on my program. He shared my book with his doctor who told him the suggested remedy would do nothing for his condition.

When this man called me September 14, he was quite happy and seemed to have a very deep sense of emotional appreciation. He told me his ALT and his AST were normal for the first time since he had been having his blood tested. His doctor wrote him a letter, which he read to me over the phone. The doctor very eloquently stated that, having been educated in the way that he was and knowing this man's condition, he knew what the outcome would be. To have the man's condition turn around in eight months was something unbelievable to the doctor.

Because of the doctor's unique relationship with this man, he was actually able to see and document what was going on, and be able to believe it. I say believe it, because so many doctors across this country tell people who use my program with success that they are having a "spontaneous remission." The doctor told him "I think I'm going to have to re-educate myself because I don't think this was a spontaneous remission."

The doctor recommended another biopsy to examine the cirrhosis and the patient refused. We do know that the liver panel is normal for the first time and he feels better now than he has for at least ten years.

Lloyd

**Another Doctor Agrees!**

Dear Lloyd,

I have been taking the Natcell frozen thymus for about two months now along with the reishi mushroom and milk thistle. I also take 6000 mg's of Vitamin C and 400 mg's of lipoic acid a day. In addition, I take four ounces of aloe in the morning and four at night. The biggest difference is in the way I feel, no more sick feeling and upset stomach with no appetite.

The doctor and his assistant are very supportive of me doing this treatment, if you can believe that!

Thanks in advance,<br>Marilyn

## Challenging Medical Model

Hello, Lloyd,

I thought since we were unable to speak on the phone, I would let you know a little about the type of care I give. Most in my chiropractic profession perform spinal adjustments, as I did for years, to affect the muscle and stimulate the nerve. This type of adjustment works only because it affects the nerve function indirectly, thus allowing the body to function at a higher level and heal itself.

This type of care is cutting edge, and it has begun to grow rapidly throughout the profession. Currently, I am one of three doctors who utilize this technique, known as the Torque method, using Toggle Recoil.

I must congratulate you and recognize you for challenging the medical model. As we know, this model is set up to profit specific individuals and groups, ignoring any other options no matter how well they might work.

This is what I do every day of my life, because I realize that the third leading cause of death in this country is conventional medicine. I believe conventional medicine is killing more people than AIDS, handguns, and traffic fatalities combined. This is happening in part because of the continuing attitude you and I run into continuously from the medical establishment.

However, the good news is that the American people are realizing this slowly, and last year they visited more alternative care providers than medical providers. The ones we really need to convince are the people, as I believe only a small fragment of the medical establishment would even listen to what we have to say. They just have too much time and money invested and too much to lose.

Thankful to people like you,<br>Clarence L.

## Knowledge Is A Powerful Weapon

Dear Lloyd,

Thank you again for your book. You went through so much also! You spoke of your descent into "Hell" when the tractor fell on you. Yes, I know exactly what you mean. When I fell down the steps and went into a coma, life was never the same afterward. Dramatic differences, eh?

I have rapid and frequent fluctuations in my energy/moods. Is this normal? I am watching everything that I put into my body, i.e. the quality of water, food, supplements, stress levels, etc. I am at a plateau right now.

I am drinking 4 shots of wheat grass per day. It makes me very nauseous. Maybe detoxifying? And I'm still doing yoga as much as possible. I nap every afternoon because I'm dead tired with mental fogs. Ammonia levels? My appetite is decreasing, and I am losing weight. I think my viral load may be decreasing.

I've been told to apply for disability due to my head injury and coma, loss of hearing, smell and taste, depression, recent addiction recovery and hepatitis C activity. I was told that people with less going on than I have qualify. Working makes me VERY tired. I don't WANT to be on disability, I want my normal life back, and

I need to pay for all this stuff to make me BETTER! Is there anything you can tell me to help regarding disability?

I know you are a busy man, and I apologize for asking you these questions, but I do not know of anyone else who is more knowledgeable about this subject, ESPECIALLY doctors! Knowledge is a powerful weapon, eh?

Ciao, fondly,
Leona


Dear Leona,

I do not know where disability payments will get you; it does not pay enough to accomplish anything. The medicine they may provide will not help much.

You need to get started on at least part of my program to get some drive-for-life back. Even just by taking dandelion root tea, you can get a lot of the toxins out of your blood so you are not so tired. Hyssop tea will give you more energy. Milk thistle will work wonders. Wheat grass may be great, but it isn't going to cure hepatitis C. Also 200 mg of lipoic acid three times a day and 400 mcg of selenium together can help you a lot.

We need to perk you up so that when you are working as a waitress, you dazzle people and they give you bigger tips! Your rapid fluctuation in energy levels is certainly not uncommon with hepatitis C. Of course, the doctors don't always agree, but I hear it every day. People on my program have a great improvement in this area.

In good health,
Lloyd

## Does My Brother Have A Chance With Life?

Dear Lloyd,

I just ordered your book for my brother who has hepatitis C. He visited the doctor today, who told him was just at the beginning of the third stage. My brother is in his 30s, and the doctor says he has a good 14 years left to live. I have 5 brothers and 1 sister, and we were all devastated! We have not told our parents yet.

Does my brother still have a chance with life? I'm not quite sure what kind of medicine he'll be taking. Although I just found out today he has to take some pills and injections in his stomach and thighs. Please email me; we're all very desperate.

Leonore

Dear Leonore,

I believe it would be best if he stopped taking interferon and Ribavirin. These drugs cause side effects, and it is beyond belief what can happen. I have spoken with over 30,000 people who have used these drugs and the have drugs failed. I believe he will experience great relief from following my program.

Lloyd

## Should I Really Be Worried?

Dear Lloyd,

I found out that I have hep C in November 2000; it is now the end of December. My doctor wants me to wait for the new treatment coming out soon pegylated interferon. I am doing nothing now.

My first ALT was 83 and AST was 65 on 3/30/00. I was supposed to come back three months later and get retested. I did, and the second test on 10-27-00 showed ALT was 197 and AST was 149.

I had a biopsy done 11/27/00, and it said chronic active hepatitis C with periportal fibrosis. The microscopic part said "sections reveal infiltration of the lymphocytes in the portal triads, some lymphocytes migrate into the hepatocytes. Lymphoid aggregates are seen. Hepatic lobules are focally infiltrated by lymphocytes. The sinusoids exhibit the hyperplasic Kupffer cells and a few lymphocytes. Tricrome staining demonstrates periportal fibrosis."

I feel fine and have no symptoms. I do not know what to expect. I am scared and confused. My doctor says to wait, but he cannot say for how long. I recently spent a lot of money seeing a nutritionist, and took lots of vitamins for a month or so. It gave me diarrhea and I quit.

Please tell me how bad I am. What does my biopsy mean? How high will the numbers get on blood work? Should I really be worried? I ordered your book today. Please respond to me. I have no one to talk to that understands, and I sure don't understand.

Thanks,<br>Catharine

Dear Catharine,

Number one, do not use pegylated interferon. It does not work. I have had some people thank me a lot for warning them about what a sham this new drug is and the damage that it can do. It is being hyped to increase the value of the maker's stock. Some doctors know it the pegylated interferon does not work any better than the original interferon, and some don't. It was designed to help reduce side effects, but it is exactly the same as the original interferon, only time-released. It does make people sicker for some reason. Save yourself, and forget that poison! I have had experience with people who used it and it failed. Has your doctor? The company news releases do not tell the whole truth.

Your liver biopsy is not that bad. If you follow what is in my book, you can reverse your condition. I have had people with cirrhosis reverse it, and people who are supposed to be dead, are now celebrating.

Naturopaths, for the most part, do not know what they are doing. I have seen a lot of them and shared the speaking stage with a few. I am overwhelmed by how uneducated these people are about hepatitis C, among other issues. Vitamins are not the answer here.

People who do what I did have the best results in the shortest time. People who alter my program do not do as well. The remedy in *Triumph Over Hepatitis C* works, and you feel good while you are doing it.

In good health,
Lloyd

## Don't Wait For The Doctors

Dear Lloyd,

If there is anything in any of the emails I send you that you feel would be of any assistance to anyone else, please feel free to edit and add them to your message board.

You were gracious enough to send me your book. I read it and decided that I cannot wait for the doctors and their "new" form of interferon. The old form is too dangerous for me, so why wouldn't the new form be the same?

Back in June, my viral load was 590,000, my AST 49, and my ALT 60. Well, my doctor called me this afternoon to let me know that he had mailed me the results of the blood work that he ordered for me two weeks or so ago. Now, December 28, my viral load is over 1,000,000. He didn't give me the other results. I will wait for the mail. This is what I get for doing what the doctors say and waiting for their drugs.

I still have not received a disability check, so I have been unable to get any herbs. However, on Christmas Eve, a friend stopped by with a plain brown paper bag in her hands. She gave it to me and said, "Merry Christmas." I stuck my hand in the paper bag and felt plastic baggies. This angel of a woman smiled as I pulled out two bags of milk thistle seeds and dandelion root. Needless to say, there are two pots on the stove right now with weird tea in them.

All I can say is, for the sake of your own life DON'T WAIT FOR THE DOCTORS. It can kill you while you're waiting.

Nancy

Dear Nancy,

I would wait for the grave before I would use pegylated interferon. Just last night, I received a rewarding email from one of my clients. In the last three months, his viral load has dropped from 521,520 to 119,250. Blood test on file

That could be you!<br>Lloyd

## Hostility, Arrogance from HMO Doctor

Hello Lloyd:

I am a member of Kaiser Permanente HMO through my workplace. They diagnosed me last August with hep C. My AST was 49 and ALT was 97, indicating liver inflammation. The PCR test was 437000 IU/ml; apparently that's the viral load.

Along with your book, I've also been reading *The Hep C Handbook* by Matthew Dolan. His statistics indicate that under 1 million is considered low. So, after four months of following the recommendations in your book, I asked to be tested again. The doctor would only allow the ALT test, which came back as 122 u/l, a small increase in this enzyme's presence in my blood sample.

I contacted my doctor, because I had asked to be tested for viral load. In speaking with her, I was amazed at the level of hostility and arrogance when I tried to query her. I wanted the PCR test, but she would not okay it.

Reading Dolan's book, I see he raises doubts about the ALT and AST tests as absolute indicators of hep C progression. And he also mentions that the PCR tests are expensive, and many hospitals are averse to multiple testing. So my take is that my doctor is more cost-conscious, it being an HMO.

Interestingly, when I told her I was taking herbs and vitamin supplements that other people had claimed worked, she became even more hostile, saying "It's all rubbish; name a journal where these results have been published," et cetera.

I was blown away by her arrogance. Also, she said that my viral load was high, but according to what I've read, it's low. I am going to give her a break. She's probably overworked and stressed out working for an HMO. Also she's a general practitioner, and she probably doesn't have the time to keep up on developments in liver pathology research.

Anyway, the long and short of it is that she won't give me the PCR test. After that phone call, I started going through the yellow pages looking for labs. I each one I called that I wanted to be tested for hep C viral load and could they do it? "Yes," they said. "Can I come in and pay you cash?" "No–you need a doctor's request." What is this–Catch 22?

Conventional wisdom, as propagated through the medical establishment or the government, has always been highly suspect to my mind, and this little episode reminds me of your comment about Dylan's tune, "Political World."

I continue on your program, and I am attempting to find a private source for PCR testing. If you can recommend any labs in the Bay area, that would be great. If not, I will continue researching.

I've got faith in your program and the innate healing powers of the body. We're not little statistical samples; we're the product of an incredible life force.

Thanks,<br>Paul

Dear Paul,

What you describe is very much the norm with Kaiser. The viral load test is often rejected unless you agree to do the interferon. The attitude against alternative medicine is almost universal, either for lack of knowledge or money. It is an unfortunate situation.

I have a doctor who faxes me the prescription for the test I want. I go to the lab of my choice, the test is performed, and the doctor faxes the results. Then, I set up a payment plan with the lab. It's that simple.

Did the doctor tell you to fast before the test? If not, the results are worthless. By the way, a liver panel, which costs $33.00, does many more tests than one. It is a scam for money.

I would like to put your email on my message board to show people just how rebellious doctors still are. I suggest you read the chapter on albumin in my book, which is about a doctor back in the 1840s, who tried to tell his fellow physicians to wash their hands. It is an example of just how arrogant, unchangeable, and inflexible doctors are, and have been for hundreds of years.

Lloyd

## Docs Were Not Giving Us Any Hope

Dear Lloyd,

We received your book in the mail last Wednesday along with many supplements. My husband and I are nearly finished reading it. Wow, it was so inspiring! I just wanted to extend our thanks and appreciation to you.

A large part of the reason my husband was in denial was due to the fact the docs were not giving us any hope. You have completely changed his entire outlook on hepatitis C and how we can deal with this. He has not been this positive for many, many months. Now he's acting like a different person. For that, I thank you from the bottom of my heart.

He has been religiously taking the following:

Milk thistle 400 mg 3x day
Lipoic acid 200 mg 3x day

Selenium 400 mg daily
Licorice 500 mg 2x day
Dandelion 500 mg 3x day
Cat's claw 250 mg 2x day
Vitamin C 5000 mg 2x day
Reishi mushroom 510 mg 2x day
Alfalfa 2x day
Colostrum 900 mg daily
Dandelion tea, 1 qt, daily, with 2 lemons juiced
Natcell Thymus 1 vial every other day
Aloe from whole plant 4 to 8oz daily

I would appreciate your opinion on any changes we need to make. Also, how long should he wait before he has his next set of labs done? He swears that he already feels more energy, and he is less fatigued, all in less than a week! I have noticed he is not so edgy.

Lloyd, thank you again. I truly believe you are an angel sent to us from God. Look forward to hearing from you soon.

Samantha

## "What is Thymus?" Doc Asks and "Pooh-Poohs" Milk Thistle

Dear Lloyd,

Thank you so much for your truly inspirational book! I received it yesterday and finished reading it this a.m. I share your opinion of western doctors and have had many a nightmare dealing with them. I decided early on when I was diagnosed with hepatitis C that interferon and MD's were not in my best interest, nor were they a positive approach to overcoming the trials and tribulations of this disease.

I started immediately on a program change that affected not only my diet, but also my general outlook on life. My mother-in-law found some amazing information on thymus and its results that were achieved with hepatitis C. Mind you, before my mother-in-law found out about thymus, I was in bad shape with the normal hepatitis C-related symptoms!

Within two weeks of taking "the complete thymus formula," I felt 100% better! Then, I went to my gastroenterologist to see if this formula was suitable for my condition. He said, "Thymus? What is thymus? What do you mean thymus?" I was shocked, and replied, "You don't know?" Then he said, "I don't know about any 'thymus'. The only herb I've heard of being used for hepatitis C is milk thistle and that hasn't been proven to do anything, really."

Needless to say, I don't talk to this doctor much except to get blood work tests done. I am extremely excited about starting your program. Thanks again.

Sincerely,
Bernard

## A Basic Distrust Of Medicos

Hello Lloyd,

I just finished reading your book. I have had similar nightmares with the medical community. I was also lucky enough to have a basic distrust of medicos, and so I decided to do nothing until I found something that made sense.

You at least have made yourself disease-free, and you have a similar distrust and disgust for what the medical profession passes off as treatment, which is really torture.

Thanks,<br>Bobby

## I Want Dr. Right!

Hello Lloyd,

Want to hear a funny story? At present my doctor is Dr. Wong (nice person, but kind of clueless). After three visits with this doctor, I was frustrated with him and mentioned that "I no longer want Dr. Wong, I want Dr. Right!" Anyway, Mr. Wright, I know you aren't a doctor, but I thought it was funny.

I am 37 years old and was diagnosed with hepatitis C three months ago. Dr. Wong (there's that name again) told me to take a multi-vitamin and not to worry about it. He forgot to mention to get a vitamin without iron, or alas, he doesn't even know. I suspect the latter to be true.

He ordered a biopsy, which I had six weeks ago. He asked if I could donate a small piece of my liver for a research study which I was told would be taken after they made sure there was enough for my biopsy results. Hey, guess what! Yes, you are right. On the biopsy, it was mentioned twice that the sample of liver was too small for conclusive results (as to whether I have bridging fibrosis or not). Just a little tidbit I thought I would throw in for your reading entertainment.

The results of the biopsy showed I have fibrosis and piecemeal necrosis (less than 50%). My doctor then said, after patting me on the shoulder, treatment, treatment, treatment, interferon, interferon, interferon! And then he popped off in his SUV to the coffee shop for a nice cup of tea and a Danish.

Why am I telling you all this? I want to know exactly what supplements to take, how many to take and how often to take them. I plan to go to Mexico for three months and would like to be as healthy as possible and boost my immune system as best I can before I go. I plan to eat as healthy as possible and take any supplements that will improve my prognosis. But, alas, I am in the dark as to what I have to take to give myself the best possible chance, which foods to eat, etc.

I read your book last night, and was encouraged that there is a possible cure for myself with alternative medicine. Because I'll be camping for three months without a freezer, I'll be taking the capsules instead of the live cell thymus.

I need to know what to take along for a three-month supply of supplements, along with a list of foods to eat, and what to drink. If you do this, I'll buy you a big Mexican hat. I'm willing to give alternative medicine a shot. It seems more natural and less chemical.

Yours sincerely,
Andy

P.S. Why was six scared of seven?
Because seven eight nine!


## Desperate To Get The Iron Out

Dear Lloyd!

It's me again. Don't you know I just got word from the doctor that he wants to do a liver biopsy before he will do a phlebotomy! Can you believe it? Of course you can.

I have called several other places to get rid of this blood but nobody will do it. Please, do you have any suggestions? I'm getting desperate. Do any of the people that write you or call have any suggestions? I really need to get this iron out.

HELP! As ever,
Victor

Dear Victor,

All a doctor really needs to know to prescribe blood-letting is that it will not hurt you and that a general blood test that includes platelet count is all that is necessary.

Also, there must be a general doctor around who would do this. You might try a private nurse who would do it.

Let me know what happens.

Lloyd

## What To Do About "The Doctor End of Things"

Dear Lloyd,

I am 47 years old, and I feel great. Sometimes I do feel pain near my liver when I take too many energy herbs. (I work construction, and at my age, I need all the energy I can get). I found out I have hepatitis C during a routine physical. I am supposed to see a liver specialist. After reading your book, I am not sure what to do about the doctor end of things.

I have taken herbs for about nine years. I have started taking milk thistle, licorice, alfalfa, dandelion, cat's claw. My AST was 35; my ALT was 65. Please advise me if you have time.

Dick

179

## Lloyd speaks at U.S. Berkeley–Notes Medical Malaise

Dear Dick,

The items you are taking are good, but you need to add a few items.

Natcell Thymus (1 vial every other day), Pure Synergy, vitamin B, vitamin C taken to tolerance, selenium 400 mcg., and lipoic acid 200 mg. 3 times per day. These will help a lot.

Going to see a gastroenterologist will result in the following;

1. Liver biopsy, (required before interferon treatment);

2. They will attempt to make you believe that interferon is the only way; and

3. They will tell you there is no other way. I went through all this six years ago.

I hear about what goes on from the thousands of phone calls and emails I receive each week. I spoke at the University of California at Berkeley yesterday at a hepatitis C meeting and found similar problems with some of those doctors.

The social anthropologists at Berkeley invited me to speak because they believe that the United States is in a backward, money-motivated medical malaise equal to the Dark Ages when it comes to the treatment of virus. MD's are great if you've got a bone jutting out of your body, but give them a chance to treat virus, and they will take every cent you or your insurance company have, and you will still be sick.

In good health,<br>Lloyd

## Quality of Care, Or Rather Lack of It

Dear Lloyd,

I have had hepatitis C since 1968. Dr. G. tells me that I have 50% of my liver function left. My friend told me about your web site. I am considering alternatives to medical treatment. I have been very dissatisfied with my endocrinologist's quality of care, or rather the lack of it. I am looking forward to reading your book.

Thanx,<br>Benjamin

## Variations on the Diagnosis Theme

Dear Lloyd,

I just received your book today one hour before calling and getting my latest lab results back. I've known I've had hepatitis C since 1993, and I have been seeing a doctor. He kept telling me my levels were in the high normal range.

Not knowing much, I took his word that I needn't worry. Well, I recently had an appointment with a new doctor, and he wondered why I hadn't had a liver biopsy or started interferon. I told him my previous doctor said it wasn't necessary. He did more blood work and said to call him in two weeks. Since that appointment, I found your web site and have read everything in it. Thank God I found you. I was ready to start interferon.

Angalena

Dear Angalena,

I am happy that you found me as well. Interferon is poison and generally does not work. If you do as I did, you will improve; and if you do it long enough, you will get well.

Lloyd

## Can't Concentrate; On the Verge of Tears; Please Tell Me What I Should Take

Dear Lloyd,

Please forgive any rambling (bad brain fog and two toddlers). I ordered your book and tried to read it, but just can't concentrate long enough to figure out what to do.

I'm having blood drawn this coming Saturday, so I have no numbers yet. I was diagnosed with hepatitis C last summer. I know you say you're not a doctor, but could you please tell me what I should take first, in order to begin to function again? Sorry, I'm on the verge of tears right now.

Thanks,
Lorraine

Dear Lorraine,

Do not take interferon. Do not take Peg-Intron. You need to do what is in my book. It is a simple book to read.

You can call me toll free at (877) 676-1615.

You have nothing to worry about except letting the doctors try to kill you.

Lloyd

## Doc's Revelation: Nothing Left Except Possibly Alternative Medicine

Dear Lloyd,

Our daughter is very bad. She has taken interferon and her test results following it showed no improvement. Instead, she got worse. She is now starting that treatment over again, along with some by-mouth medication. Doctors tell her that if this doesn't help, nothing is left except possibly alternative medicine.

Ann

## Specialist Versus Regular Doctor

Dear Lloyd,

My ALT was 42 at my first blood test. It was 56 after 6 months. I've been taking the herbal supplements since August 2000. My last blood test in November showed everything in the normal range. My ALT was 22, amazing!

I told my specialist what I had been taking, and he told me to keep taking the milk thistle. My regular doctor told me I was wasting my money. The specialist told me to come back in a year.

Thank you for turning me and others on to these herbal supplements. I still wonder if the Natcell Thymus would cure this completely like it did for you. I know everybody is different; the only way to find out is just to try it.

Thanks again,
Beatrice

## Doctors And Insurance

Good morning, Lloyd,

I am TJ from Minnesota. We spoke on the phone last Saturday morning. I am going to start on your remedy plan. I have my blood tests, which I will send to you with my mail order so we have a starting base. I also had a genotype test run, which was inconclusive (according to my GI).

The PCR test was positive, but came with no quantitative asset (viral load). I called my gastroenterologist to have the genotype and RNA by PCR tests redone. He said that the tests are unreliable, expensive, and he can't order them to track some kind of alternative therapy medicine. Also, he told me to call Health Partners (my insurance provider) if I want to dispute this.

I am not sure what to do. These tests are important. Please help me. I want to start the remedy soon.

Thank you,<br>TJ

Dear TJ,

Most insurance providers will provide tests for a while. Some will demand that you do interferon at some point, or else they will discontinue payment for tests.

Your doctor or insurance company is jerking you around. I think you should read your contract with the insurance company to see what your rights are. I paid cash for my tests, so whatever alternatives to medical insurance you can think of, I would do them.

Also, I would like to print this email on my message board so people who do not have a clue how bad off our insurance companies are can get an idea. Keep trying,

Lloyd

## Just Wait For A Better Cure

Dear Lloyd,

Last week, my husband went in for his annual checkup with his specialist concerning his hepatitis C. Of course, his blood levels were up a bit, but the real reason we went at this time, was to talk about your book and the therapy that you were on. I have had my husband on the milk thistle now for about three weeks.

The doctor basically told us to be careful, which I thought he would say. We told him that my husband COULD NOT handle the interferon anymore because of all the side effects, especially the mental part.

The doctor's advice was to get another liver biopsy. Thank God, the last time we had his liver checked it was in pretty good shape.

The doctor also said that herbs are NOT proven to work, which I knew he would say. So, we are just supposed to sit back until they find a cure or a better treatment. His advice was just to wait!  I don't feel comfortable with that at all! Please help with some advice. Any would be good!

Thank you so much,
Shirley


Dear Shirley,

If you read my book, you will see they told me basically the same thing, except that I only had 3 to 5 years to live. They also told me to wait for something new to come along.

Should the United States have waited any longer to contain Hitler? Should I have waited any longer for a cure? If I had, I would be dead. I know some people who, back in

185

the 1970s, were waiting for the price of real estate to come down before they bought a home. They're still waiting.

So what do you think you should do?

Lloyd

## Doc Too Stupid To Look Into Natural Medicine

Lloyd,

The doctor just called me here at work to talk to me about the pilot program of Amantadine and Ribavirin. I asked him about my ALT, and it was 58 compared to the 89 it had been. He said it had gone as high as 100. Also, some of the other values are down.

They finally are going to send me a copy of the results. I said, "So the figures are down?" The doctor said, "Yes." "I guess alternative meds do work," I replied. He said, "What are you taking, the milk thistle?" I told him I was taking that and some other things. Anyway, he said it would not eliminate the virus, only protect my life.

Arty

Dear Arty,

Well, perhaps you should give him something to talk about. Do the program, get well, and tell him he was wrong and that he is responsible for millions of deaths because he was too stupid to look into natural medicine.

Lloyd

## No Tests Exist?

Dear Lloyd,

I contacted my doctor's office about my viral load. They said it's over a million and that's all they can tell me. I

186

asked for a prescription to have a test done that is specific, not a range. Their reply was that "over one million" is extremely high, and no tests exist for a viral load that high.

The doctor said that if such a test exists, he's unaware of it, but he would write the prescription if I knew what the test was. Are they right? Or does the test exist and they just don't know about it? Thanks,

Marsha

Dear Marsha,

I have tests results from hundreds of people who are over a million and up to 102,000,000, which is the highest viral load I've seen. I get them every week that are 5,000,000, 10,000,000, 32,000,000. So you see, over one million is not uncommon.

If your doctor doesn't know the proper tests for hepatitis C, how does he expect to treat it? I don't know what to say. Perhaps he should call the company that does the tests and ask them what he should be doing.

Lloyd

Dear Lloyd,

That is really scary. Now I'm not sure what to do. Of course, every time you change doctors the first thing they want is a $200.00 visit.

Maybe I can find a way to teach this doctor how to do at least the viral load test. What is really scary is I went to this doctor because he's supposed to be a hepatitis C expert.

Thanks for the information,<br>Marsha

## At Last, Support From a Doctor

Dear Lloyd,

Was at my gastroenterologist's office today, and I had your book in hand once again. He took an interest in it. First thing he wanted to see was your blood work (I had the page marked). After he saw that, he started flipping through the book and reading portions of it.

He was quite amused at some of your humor and laughed out loud a couple times. He especially liked your reaction as you saw the length of the needle when you had a liver biopsy done. He laughed and said, "Nancy, I would need one that long for you." He spent enough time with your book to get a good idea of what you have done and are doing. His response to me was, "Nancy, we cannot use my medicine for you. Do what this guy tells you to do!"

I am very free in giving your name and web site to any and all I encounter with this disease. So, my friend, I am on my way. I know you wish me luck. I know this will work. By the way, I have now lost 40 lbs, a really good start.

Take care,
Nancy

## Virus-Free...With a High Count?

Dear Lloyd,

My husband has hepatitis C, and he has been on the interferon and Rebetrol for 52 weeks. After he was done with his treatment, the doctor said he was virus free.

Now he took another test (hep C viral RNA by PCR, Quantitative). The doctors are now saying this is a test they do 3 times: one time in the beginning of treatment (don't know what the count was), one time in the middle (the

188

count was below 1,000), and one time at the end of treatment, his count now being at 15,000. They said they'd never seen this happen before.

We are puzzled. How can he be virus-free and now have a count this high? We told them to do the test over. They wanted my husband to go to a liver specialist, but we do not feel good about this doctor, and we are looking for alternatives. What do you think? Any input would be greatly appreciated.

Sincerely,<br>Sandra

Dear Sandra,

More than 99% of all people who are cleared from the virus with interferon have it come back in 6 to 12 months. If your doctor said he'd never seen this before, he is either stupid, living in the dark ages, or a liar, or all three.

The number 15,000 is not really that high. I have people who have viral loads over 60,000,000.

If you want to get well, now is the time to do the remedy in *Triumph Over Hepatitis C.*

In good health,<br>Lloyd

## Docs Quick To Recommend "Painless" Interferon

Dear Lloyd,

I find your book fascinating, although I am still a little overwhelmed with my recent diagnosis and the amount of conflicting information being slung at me from every direction.

What I have noticed, which was also confirmed in your book, is that the medical doctors seem quick to recommend interferon. My doctor told me today that the side effects of the drug were "blown way out of proportion," and that many of his patients hadn't even felt a thing.

Anyway, my viral load was 350,000 (does that sound right?) and I'm scheduled to have a biopsy in a week, after which I assume it will be recommended that I start this "painless" interferon treatment. I have already decided to try everything else before I resort to that treatment.

I look forward to hearing from you. Thanks for the light at the end of this very black tunnel!

Bernie

## I Don't Have to Die

Dear Lloyd,

I just finished your book. I loved it! Now I think, "Great, I don't have to die." Of course, my doc thinks you are a quack, but I want to show him the Yale study that was mentioned on the cover of your book. Thank you for giving us all much needed help. God bless.

Janice

Dear Janice,

Most doctors are negative about my program, but I haven't had one call me a quack yet. Perhaps your doctor should go to my web site and read about all the people who are doing far better on my program than they did on the interferon/Ribavirin combo. I will attempt to attach the Yale article onto this email and also one from Russia.

In good health,<br>Lloyd

P.S. The article from Russia is on a different computer, so maybe you can read it on my message board. It is also about thymus.

**Physician Who Has Hep C Becomes Medical Heretic**

Dear Lloyd,

I attended the Cancer Care conference at Universal this past summer, heard your lecture, purchased your book, and met you briefly after your lecture. Although I am a physician, I have been a medical heretic for years and practice using only non-toxic therapies, such as chelation, bio-oxidative, orthomolecular doses of IV vitamins, etc.

Just as you once did, I also have hepatitis C. Strangely enough, I had hepatitis B for over 30 years. It had always been HBV S-Ag negative, HBV S-Ab positive, and I had mild elevations in my transaminases. Furthermore, I tested negative for hepatitis C at one point, although I do not recall when that was.

Last November, I was shocked to learn that my enzymes had climbed to between 100 and 200, but that I was HBV S-Ab negative and still HBV S-Ag negative. When, by February, my transaminases had climbed to the 500 range, I checked and found that I was still negative for HBV, but positive HCV! I guess I do believe in pleomorphism.

I immediately adopted a 100% raw food, vegan diet and began using large amounts of silymarin and other herbs. By August, my enzymes were down to under 100 again. I now eat about a 90% raw diet. I thoroughly enjoyed your lecture and book, and I am very anxious to get started on the protocol you advocate. Please advise!

Thank you,
Thom Lodi

## High Price for Doc's Supplement

Dear Lloyd,

Do you carry an artichoke supplement? A doctor told me this is great stuff for the liver, but he wants over $100 for a small bottle. I just don't have that kind of money. I can barely afford the milk thistle, cat's claw, dandelion root, licorice root, vitamin E and thymus.

Casey

## Read Your Book in Under an Hour

Dear Lloyd,

Just received your book and started on Natcell Thymus. Read your book in under an hour. It was great, and I identified with you immediately about MD's, insurance companies, and pharmaceutical profits. Really enjoyed your candid and honest style!

Thx again,
Dave

## I No Longer Believe in Transplant Team

Lloyd,

My husband was diagnosed in 1998 with hep C and cirrhosis. We did find the herb milk thistle, and he had been taking it. The doctors kept saying that he should feel sicker based on his blood work. He did have a spot on the liver at that time, but they dismissed it as nothing. Now, my husband has liver cancer and is taking tons of medications.

The tumor was 4.7 cm by the time they found it. Apparently, it was there all along, but they dismissed it because his alpha feta protein levels had never been elevated.

He has undergone 2 chemoembolization treatments since August. I am losing him, I can tell. We were able to find a potential partial-liver donor, but the transplant team is really dragging its feet. They keep saying there are scheduling problems. I am really scared. My brother is willing to start testing (blood work, etc.) as a donor today, but the team says it will be sometime after February 1. Every day, the risk of the cancer spreading is there.

John is not just my husband, but also my best friend. We've been married for 19 years. We are more in love today than ever, and it was that way before the cancer diagnosis. We worked together for years in our own business before losing his son (my stepson). I feel like I'm losing my best friend. Do you have any advice? I'm really scared.

I believe in God and pray, but I feel I need to try anything I can to save his life. I'm sorry I haven't tried sooner, but I believed in the transplant team. I no longer believe in them.

Thank you,
Pam

## Doc Has His Brain Twisted

Dear Lloyd,

I am an HCV patient and currently take some of the products that you talk about in your book. One of my doctors recommends that I take a multi-vitamin that includes 55,000 IU of vitamin A daily. I feel that this is too much. What is your opinion? I also take EPA/DHA (essential fatty acids from cold water fish). What is your opinion on this?

Please reply,
Laura

Dear Laura,

An amount of 55,000 IU of vitamin A is ridiculous. The man has his brain twisted. Nothing above normal vitamin A is advisable. And even that is sometimes too much. There may be something about your particular case I am unaware of, but vitamin A is generally not good for liver disease. The other items you mentioned sound fine.

Lloyd

## Fluid Pills That Do Not Work

Hey, Lloyd,

We just ordered the Natcell Thymus. Your book is very funny (kind of sick humor, but we know where you are coming from!). The MD's answer to bloating (fluid retention in the abdomen) is fluid pills, and they do not work. What has helped everyone you know get rid of that? The doctor is of little to no help, and Ben is in stage 4 cirrhosis.

Sheri and Ben

Dear Sheri and Ben,

The reason fluid pills do not work is that the fluid is lymphatic fluid and not water retention. This is often misdiagnosed and has led to death for some people I have met. It needs to be manually removed. The best way to stop it is live cell thymus and live cell liver.

Lloyd

## Doc Gave Me a Death Sentence And
## A Magazine Featuring Naomi Judd

Dear Lloyd,

Just received your book; it's great. Like most, I had a great hepatologist that gave me a death sentence and a magazine, with Naomi Judd on the cover, to read about this disease. He hands them out in his waiting room like those magazines we read as kids in waiting rooms, "Highlights Juniors" where we found the hidden things in the pictures.

Well, the magazine on hep was just about the same: all mazes and questions, with no answers at the bottom of the pages or anything. After finding out I had the genotype 1a and doing research, I felt the interferon combo was just a waste of time, money and sanity.

I wanted to let you know about this report in my newspaper magazine section today. Parade Magazine Advocate Newspaper, Stamford, CT., Intelligence Report. "David Satcher, the U.S. Surgeon General, is short on postage stamps. Why should this concern you? Well, Dr. Satcher wanted to mail a letter to every U.S. household warning of a potential health danger. (The last time a Surgeon General did this, it was C. Everett Koop, and the danger was AIDS.) Satcher wrote the letter, but his budget doesn't have enough money left to mail it. So we'll tell you about it here. The health danger is a liver disease known as hepatitis C." The story goes on to tell you bits of info and sends you to a web site.

Can you believe this? I'm sure you can, but it just goes to prove your theory on the sad state of affairs this country is in, health-wise. If you know of any doctors in this area willing to treat this disease, could you let me know? I live in Greenwich, CT., and all I can find are uptight doctors only willing to fight it with drugs that won't help.

Thank you for your book.

Vickie

## Comment by Lloyd:

The following report, written by the executive director of the Hepatitis C Support Project in Santa Barbara, CA, has information relating to the above letter. The report is also posted on my web site message board:

July 8, 2001

The Grave Threat of HCV

By Kathy Lusting, Executive Director,
Hepatitis C Support Project, Santa Barbara, CA

The 106th Congress ended in October with one major victory and one major setback. We got the first piece of major federal legislation with a title for hepatitis C virus (HCV). The HCV title is in the Children's Health Care Act of 2000, which often authorizes the Center for Disease Control and Prevention (CDC) to establish national surveillance of chronic hepatitis C and education programs for health-care professionals and the public. The next step is to get Congress to give the CDC money specifically for the HCV surveillance and education program.

Within the same halls of Congress, Republican and Democratic leadership joined forces to develop the Children's Health Care Act, but a planned national HCV Alert was dropped. The Commerce Committee and Surgeon General David Satcher had planned to send a letter to every American household alerting the public to the risk of HCV. Satcher had previously declared hepatitis C an epidemic and a "grave threat" to the American public's health. But when push came to shove, Satcher and the Commerce Committee backed down from sending the letter, saying it could not go out because there was no money to pay for the postage. As a result, what should have been a sincere effort at public education will probably remain on the Surgeon General's desk through the end of this presidential administration.

The letter experience–and the HCV title in the children's bill–is unfortunately characteristic of other federal responses to the hepatitis C epidemic by this administration. The Food and Drug Administration has repeatedly postponed a huge blood "look-back" program to notify people who had received blood transfusions potentially contaminated with hepatitis C virus. The look-back was launched three years ago, but the original intent of the advisory committee on blood safety and availability remains only partially implemented.

There are several other examples of this neglectful pattern. The Secretary of Health and Human Services (HHS) announced an HCV initiative in January 1998 that, in addition to launching the look-back, gave the CDC responsibility for a general public education campaign on hepatitis C. The CDC's budgets in recent years have included roughly $1 million a year for public education on this disease. However, there is little evidence of any of their general public-education efforts. A pilot public-education program that the CDC launched in Washington, D.C. and Chicago in fiscal year 1999 was discontinued in fiscal year 2000, after spending only $70,000. And recent work plans have mentioned only education initiatives targeted to high-risk groups.

The Department of Veterans Affairs (VA) announced a high-profile initiative on hepatitis C in January 1999, in response to an estimated infection rate of 8 to 10 percent among veterans. **(Comment by Lloyd: Vietnam veterans have a 65 percent infection rate.)** Congress followed by providing the VA an additional $350 million for hepatitis C testing and treatment in fiscal year 2000. While 179,000 veterans have already tested positive in the VA, the VA had stated it expected to treat only 9,750 of them in fiscal year 2000. As of the end the first half of the fiscal year 2000, only 1,100 veterans had received treatment and only $39 million of its HCV funds were spent. Although the VA's commitment to this initiative seems sincere, its failure to implement it is disturbing.

The CDC also has responsibility for surveillance of infectious disease and for providing information on the incidence and prevalence of disease in the population. Despite the initiative announced by the HHS Secretary in 1998, the CDC has continued to instruct the states not to report cases of chronic infection. In doing so, they have ignored recommendations for surveillance for the Secretary's own advisory committee on blood safety and availability and from the council of state and territorial epidemiologists. Instead, the Center has continued to use estimates of prevalence from data collected in 1991, before an accurate blood test for HCV was available, and to rely on incident data from a few "sentinel counties." There is no national surveillance system that can accurately inform public health officials about the incidence of prevalence of this infectious disease in their communities.

198

I marvel at this administration's failure to notify the public or respond with effective screening or treatment initiatives. An estimated four million Americans are infected with HCV today–most of them infected before a blood test was available–and at least 70 percent of these remain unaware of their illness. A disease that is four times as prevalent as AIDS, and that is projected within the decade to kill more people each year than AIDS, seems to me to be sufficient cause for major public-education initiative.

The Secretary's advisory committee on blood safety and availability summed it up when it stated in a resolution adopted on August 25, 2000:

"The committee believes that the public has not been adequately informed of the risk factors of HCV and approximately 4 million Americans may be infected with HCV, many of whom are unaware of their infection.

"The committee feels that this poses a threat to the safety of the blood supply. Therefore, the committee recommends that the Surgeon General send a letter to all U.S. households, notifying the public about the risk factors for HCV and appropriate testing treatment options."

And on a state level, in the fall of 2000, Gov. Gray Davis signed California's first hepatitis C bill, Polanco SB–1258. The bill started off with a $7 million price tag to implement testing and education in the state of California. It was reduced to $5 million, and then went to Gov. Davis desk at 2 million. Gov. Davis reduced it to $1.5 million, with half going to veterans whom already have funds budgeted for hepatitis C. Another portion was given to the Department of Corrections to reproduce a report on hepatitis C.

Several years ago, the Department of Corrections gave back significant funds for hepatitis C because it had failed to use the monies. It is estimated that close to 50 percent of the state's incarcerated are infected with hepatitis C. The state's potentially infected will be lucky to see $500,000, which amounts to about 1 dollar a patient for testing and education.

According to the CDC, 1.8 percent (or 500,000) of Californians have been exposed to the hepatitis C virus. Many of the state's experts agree, along with insurance actuaries, that projected numbers from the CDC are low, and that they are actually closer to four percent of the population who have been exposed to HCV, or 1 in 25, with 70 percent of the infected unaware they carry the disease. This author, along with other area public health officials, last spring participated in several meetings in Sacramento with the Department of Health Services in California on a hepatitis C strategic-planning committee. This plan outlines how teaching and education shall be implemented with the state. This plan has yet to be put out in final-draft form after almost one year.

In 2000, there were approximately 16,000 people on the liver transplant list in the United States, with the majority of cases caused by complications of HCV. Only 4,500 received livers. Experts predict, knowing the natural history of this disease that the number awaiting the new livers will triple over the next 10 years, with organ donations remaining the same. It is clear to this author that, with an approximately $25,000 price tag per patient and a 37 percent success rate for treatment, that sometimes includes difficult side effects, officials are slow to begin diagnosing patients. With no state or federal funds available, many county officials and public official departments find this an overwhelming task to tackle. Patient advocates would like to see a more aggressive effort to educate the general public about risk factors in transmission routes, to encourage and provide free testing, and to establish referral in case management services.

Last week, experts on hepatitis C converged in Santa Barbara for a day-long educational event targeting health-care providers. This event was organized by the Back-to-Life Hepatitis Support Project, with co-sponsors from Santa Barbara City College's Continuing Education Department, and Santa Barbara County public health and alcohol, drug and mental health services. Clearly, the full arena of more than 100 shows the interest in, and magnitude of, this disease's impact on our health-care system. Experts referred to the hepatitis C epidemic as a tidal wave off the coast of California.

Also, last week was the first successful meeting of the Hepatitis C Task Force, which was attended by representatives from impacted agencies, health-care providers, and community-based organizations. It was held at the Santa Barbara Public Health Department. Attendees listened to speakers from other organizations that have hepatitis C educational and testing models already in place in other parts of the state. The purpose of this task force is to set off a strategic plan modeled after the state Department of Health Services plan to implement testing, education, and management of hepatitis C into existing services.

## Lack of Quality Medical Care

Dear Lloyd,

I have had hep C since 1968. Dr. Gish tells me that I have 50% of my liver function left. My friend Del told me about your web site. I am considering alternatives to medical treatment. I have been very dissatisfied with my endocrinologist's quality of care, or rather the lack of it.

I am looking forward to reading your book.

Thanx,
Gregg

## Your Positive Responses Totally Overwhelmed Me

Dear Lloyd,

I met you at the CMPC Davies Campus in San Francisco. I wanted to tell you just how much of a difference your talk and Q&A session meant to me, if only to hear from a fellow sufferer, albeit a recovered sufferer, and to get the added bonus of your positive responses to my questions. It totally overwhelmed me.

I have been asking my doctors for the last five years if the chronic diarrhea I endure could be related, and they always say no! I have had tests up the ying-yang and back, and they all come away shaking their heads: "We don't know why; take this medicine and hope for the best." Also, the bruising and the subsequent shadows these tests leave were again a question that went unanswered.

I am going to start reading your book this week, and will no doubt try the herbs you recommend. Again, thanks for your positive outlook. I hope to be one of the successful people who have beaten this insidious killer disease.

Anita

Dear Anita,

Thank you for the wonderful words. If I can be of any help, just ask.

Lloyd

## Routine Tests Missed the Hep C

Hello, Lloyd,

I have just purchased and read your book. My boyfriend was just diagnosed with hep C during a routine blood test for cholesterol. He's had many such tests, and they must have missed the hep, or not told him he had it.

I thoroughly enjoyed your book, and I will be sending on to him to read. I want to understand this so I can help him. He already takes vitamins and eats well, so this won't be too much of a change for him to begin your treatment. My question is: Is this sexually transferable or not? I find different opinions. What have you found out in your research? Thank you for wanting to help others. I understand you frustration, as with any alternative medicine.

Catherine

Dear Catherine,

I appreciate your kind words about my book. I have learned much about hep C since I first wrote about it.

Hep C is not an STD! I have approximately 30,000 clients, and most of them are married and have been for many years. Only two of the couples both have hep C, other than the ones who admit to having shared needles.

I have responded to newspaper articles that clearly confuse hep C with hep B. B is an STD. It is an entirely different virus. Hep C is a blood-borne virus, and it is extremely difficult to catch. All of my past girlfriends have been tested for hep C, and none of them have it.

Any other opinion is just plain wrong! How many doctors have 26,000 people to talk to about hep C like I do? None.

One other item to consider is that the government wants the populace to believe that hep C is a lifestyle disease, not a disease caused by the medical-establishment, which it is. This causes the populace to be less concerned, and therefore less inflamed about it. The government does not want to spend money on it like they do AIDS.

In good health,<br>Lloyd

## A Rare Exception

Good morning Lloyd

I have been treated for hep C with the conventional treatment of interferon. I have been hep C free since 1998. Each time I have to go for a blood test, I fear the worst. It would be very interested in finding out more about natural products to keep me healthy.

Thanks for any help you can give me.

Linda

Dear Linda,

I think that everyone who does interferon should do my program just to recover from its effects. It does come back, nearly every time. You are the first person out of 22,000 to email me and say that you got well using interferon. This means I am going to have to change what I normally say to everyone. I am happy to finally meet someone who made it that way. I will forward you a study you may find interesting.

Lloyd

Dear Lloyd,

Just a note to let you know that as of today I continue to be hep C free. I continue to go for blood tests every six months and I guess I'll have to do so for the rest of my life. I'm thankful to be alive and healthy!

Linda

Dear Linda,

Happy New Year! It is always a pleasure to hear from someone who is staying hep C free using the modern medical approach. You are very rare. Hopefully, I will hear the same good news from you through the next decade. Take some milk thistle and dandelion root every day.

In good health,<br>Lloyd

## BEWARE OF YOUR DOCTORS OFFICE!

The following news story concerns a female kindergarten teacher who contracted hepatitis C after undergoing gastrointestinal exams in a Brooklyn clinic. She and her husband are suing the clinic for malpractice. As reported, at least eight other patients at the clinic also contracted the illness.

Clinic Sued Over Hepatitis Outbreak

NEW YORK (AP)

A woman who contracted hepatitis C after undergoing

gastrointestinal exams in a Brooklyn clinic is suing for alleged malpractice.

Deborah Postler and her husband, Stephan, filed suit in the state supreme court in Brooklyn Monday, alleging the operators of the Bay Ridge Endoscopy and Digestive Health Center were negligent in their treatment.

Deborah Postler, a kindergarten teacher, was diagnosed with hepatitis C in May after undergoing endoscopy and colonoscopy at the clinic in March. Her husband, who also filed suit, underwent a procedure at the clinic in early April and is still being tested for disease, according to the couple's lawyer, Guy Keith Vann. Deborah Postler is being treated with several drugs, some of which have caused her hair to fall out and have left her weak, with flu-like symptoms. The Postlers are seeking unspecified damages for personal and psychological injuries.

The story was first reported by the *New York Post* and the *Daily News*.

Named in the class-action lawsuit are doctors Vincent Rovito, Maria Castellano, and Marvin Chiumento. The clinic is closed, and the doctors could not be reached for comment.

At least eight other patients of the clinic came down with hepatitis C. City health officials said the flare-up was reported May 1st by the clinic's operators, who have cooperated with an ongoing investigation. Officials have notified other patients of the clinic that they should get tested for hepatitis C, which can cause long-term damage, including cirrhosis of the liver.

**Comment By Lloyd:**

I have heard from other sources that at least 30 other

victims have been identified. One is on the treatment regimen that I document in *Triumph Over Hepatitis C*. He feels great and his hair is not falling out. There are numerous statistical errors in the above news article. BEWARE OF YOUR DOCTORS OFFICE!

## Non-Detected in Two Months!

Dear Lloyd,

My husband just learned that he contracted hepatitis C through a medical procedure few months ago. We are overwhelmed. I found your web site and would like to try your regimen. I found information confusing. There is a lot of stuff to take. I am not sure which ones will be appropriate for him. He has no symptoms yet. Does he need all or some of the products? What is the schedule for taking all of it? Some of the products you mentioned you took are tea, capsules, etc. Please clarify. I just placed an order for your book, thymus extract and milk thistle.

R.C., New York

Dear R.C.,

We spoke this morning; hopefully I answered your questions. PLEASE do not take the items the doctor's recommend. You have no idea what the stuff can do. Just to give you a clear picture of what the medical community is doing, imagine the following: Picture having a daughter. Picture her getting raped. That is a very powerful, disruptive feeling! That is how I feel when someone goes on interferon, like someone is raping my daughter. If you try it, you will know exactly what I mean.

Lloyd

Dear Lloyd,

I don't know if you remember us. My husband got the virus from Brooklyn Endoscopy Center five months ago. Just wanted to let you know the good news. When we received my husband's baseline blood work, even before thymus and other stuff, his viral load was very low. We went to the doctor just recently, and he said that the virus is on the way out. We just found out new results–it is undetectable! Thanks for your help and encouragement.

R. C., New York

**Comment by Lloyd:**

These wonderful people came to me confused by the statements and lack of statements from their doctors after being infected by a medical procedure approximately five months earlier. The preceding are some of the emails between us. There were also several phone conversations between them and me, and my assistant Aunika. The news on this man being non-detected after about two months on my program is delightful! I would like to know the condition of the unfortunate people infected at approximately the same time, who elected to follow what their doctors prescribed, interferon. I am betting money they did not have this same terrific news.

Lloyd

# *SIX*

## TREATMENT "INTERFERON'ING" WITH YOUR LIFE?

### Peg-Intron: The New "Cure"

Over the last year, I began receiving phone calls from hundreds of people who were the sickest I have encountered. These were individuals who were on trials for pegylated interferon, or time-release interferon. Peg-Intron is the exact same molecule as Intron A, except that it is time-released.

The people who used this drug on a trial basis expressed to me that if their bed was located upstairs, they had to move it downstairs because they could no longer climb the stairs. They further told me they had to hire people to care for them, giving them sponge baths, even combing their hair for them, because these patients were completely incapable of functioning. None of these people ever reported to me anything but horror. No one I spoke to became non-detected for hepatitis C.

I have heard from many people who have gone to UCLA medical facilities and were told by UCLA doctors that Peg-Intron has a 95 percent success rate. I also hear this information from people who have gone to other universities throughout the country.

At UCLA, currently they are conducting trials using Peg-Intron in combination with Rebatrol, commonly referred to as the combo treatment or Ribavirin. People going into this trial are required to sign a document stating that they will not use any herbs, including milk thistle, during their trial. This to me sounds much like using humans as guinea pigs. It is clear that the health of the individual is not what is first and foremost on the minds of these "doctors."

I recently spoke to a man who has hepatitis C and whose sister has hepatitis C. She went on the pegylated interferon and Rebatrol study, after being told she had a 95% chance of being completely cured. After she was on it, she developed a seizure disorder, lost the sight in her right eye and is now legally blind. After only ten weeks on the program, she became blind in the right eye, developed astigmatism in the left eye, she is unable to focus, and she suffers from dizzy spells. She has a tingling sensation in her tongue near the back of her throat. She also suffers recurring losses of consciousness. As if this weren't enough, she has developed hearing problems as well.

It has been said to me thousands of times by thousands of people that their doctors automatically demand a liver biopsy and force interferon on people regardless of symptoms or lack of symptoms.

Why does this happen in a civilized society? Because it is the only tool in the doctors' toolbox; it is the only thing they think they have available to use. I believe one day the use of interferon for the treatment hepatitis C will be regarded as a bigger scandal than the tobacco-industry scandal. To date, I have spoken with 12 people who have gone blind from the use of Ribavirin. I have spoken to over 35,000 people who have used interferon, and not only did it fail them, but they also experienced horrible side effects. Egotistical, single-minded, money-driven doctors are in the forefront of the lack of knowledge about hepatitis C.

Peg-Intron was created by Schering-Plough to recapture market share. A couple years ago, their patent ran out and they lost market share from 2 billion a year down to 7 hundred million. In their own words, they expect their new "Gold Standard" treatment, Peg-Intron, to recapture market share to the tune of 2.4 billion.

Hepatitis C lives just above the immune system's ability to cure it. In most cases, a good immune-system boosting program can cause one's immune system to overcome the virus. I believe there is no good reason to subject us to deadly cancer drugs for the treatment of this virus.

Even Schering-Plough knows something about this: "Alpha Interferon's, including Peg-Intron, cause fatal or life-threatening neuropsychiatric, autoimmune, isochemic and infectious disorders. Patients with worsening signs or symptoms of these conditions should be withdrawn from therapy."

Contrary to what the news releases say (reprinted below), what I see and hear is that the worse the patients get, the more pills doctors prescribe to keep them on the drug. It is considered normal for people to be taking 9 to 12 different prescriptions for painkillers, tranquilizers, and mood elevators in an attempt to keep them on the drug.

This is CRIMINAL!

Below are two news releases announcing Peg-Intron, so you can see for yourself the full impact of what I'm saying. Following the reprint of the news releases, are some of the horror stories I've received from people who have tried it.

WARNING: Read these news releases at your own risk. The information contained in it is all lies! The pharmaceutical companies have propagated this information. Peg-Intron, the most recently "new and improved" form of interferon, was created because Schering-Plough's patent ran out on Intron A. To recapture its lost market share, the Schering-Plough company came out with this new form of interferon.

I have personally helped numerous people who were using this new poison on a trial basis. As a group, they are the sickest people I have encountered to date. As time goes on and we see that this new "wonder" drug has the same miserable failure rate as interferon, you will be able to determine for yourself that it doesn't live up to its hype.

The information below was issued by Schering-Plough to announce the creation of Peg-Intron, the new generation of interferon:

NEWS RELEASE:

Schering-Plough today applied to the FDA for the right to market the next generation of the combination therapy for hepatitis C. The company filed a supplemental biologics licensing application for the right to use Peg-Intron in combination with Rebetron.

Studies found that the new combination therapy, when dosed by body weight and when patients complete the full course of treatment, reduces viral levels until undetectable in 72 percent of those treated.

Clinical trials found that Peg-Intron (pegylated alfa interferon 2b) is twice as active against hepatitis C as Intron A (standard interferon). The Peg (polyethylene glycol) molecule cloaks a medicine, hiding it from the immune system and therefore allowing the drug to remain in the body longer. This makes it more effective and reduces the body's immune reaction (side effects).

Longer action also means fewer injections. Rebetol (Ribavirin) is an antiviral drug that increases the efficacy of treatment only when combined with the action of interferon.

The current leading therapy, Schering's Rebetron, is the combination of standard interferon and Ribavirin, and is effective in approximately 40 percent of patients. The combination of pegylated interferon and Ribavirin is seen as the next leading treatment.

## Comment by Lloyd:

Several months after the Peg-Intron trials were over I, began receiving calls from people who had been involved. To reiterate, this was physically the sickest group from which I have heard. On average, they had viral loads THREE times higher than when they started. They suffered the most severe disabling effects, far worse than those caused by interferon.

Side effects may continue even after a patient stops using the drug, and I have heard from several people who feel they are permanently damaged. I am personally opposed to this so-called "cure." Let me reassure you, this "snake oil" is absolute poison. I urge you to avoid it. In my opinion, it was created to help maintain market share, because Schering-Plough's patent on interferon had run out and other companies began making it, thus creating competition for Schering-Plough. Try it if you must, but when it fails, I will be here to help you recover from the results and from hepatitis C.

As you can see from the second news release reprinted below, the FDA went on to approve Peg-Intron:

**NEWS RELEASE:**

## Enzon Announces Peg-Intron (tm) Receives FDA Approval for the Treatment of Chronic Hepatitis C; First Pegylated Interferon Approved for Marketing in the United States.

PISCATAWAY, N.J.–(BUSINESS WIRE) –Jan. 22, 2001–Enzon, Inc. (NASDAQ:ENZN) announced today that Schering-Plough Corporation (NYSE:SGP) has received U.S. Food and Drug Administration (FDA) approval for Peg-Intron (TM) (peg interferon alfa-2b) powder for injection as once-weekly mono-therapy for the treatment of chronic hepatitis C in patients not previously treated with alpha interferon who have compensated liver disease and are at least 18 years of age.

Peg-Intron is the first and only pegylated interferon approved for marketing in the United States. The product is expected to be available nationwide in early February 2001.

Peg-Intron is a longer acting form of Schering-Plough Corporation's Intron(R) A that uses proprietary PEG technology developed by Enzon. Under the Company's licensing agreement with Schering-Plough Corporation, Enzon is entitled to royalties on worldwide sales of Peg-Intron and milestone payments. This approval triggers the final milestone payment of $2 million under the licensing agreement.

"While combination therapy with alpha interferon and Ribavirin is a recognized standard of care for chronic hepatitis C, Peg-Intron mono-therapy offers an alternative to patients for whom combination therapy may be a contraindication or who are intolerant of this therapy," said John G. McHutchison, MD, medical director, liver transplantation, division of gastroenterology and hepatology, Scripps Clinic and Research Foundation, La Jolla, Calif.

"As the first pegylated interferon product approved for marketing, Peg-Intron provides a valuable addition to the therapies available to physicians for treating this serious disease," Dr. McHutchison said.

"We are pleased that our Peg technology will play such an important role in the treatment of patients afflicted with this virus," said Peter G. Tombros, Enzon's president and chief executive officer. "Schering-Plough's rapid advancement of this product to the market offers evidence of the benefits that our PEG technology may provide to compounds with delivery limitations."

Peg-Intron is administered subcutaneously once weekly for one year. The dose should be administered on the same day of each week and may be self-administered by patients.

The safety and efficacy of Peg-Intron has been demonstrated in a randomized, controlled clinical study involving 1,219 adult patients with chronic hepatitis C who were not previously treated with alpha interferon.

The study compared Peg-Intron (0.5, 1.0 or 1.5 mcg/kg) administered subcutaneously once weekly to Schering-Plough's Intron(R) A (interferon alfa-2b, recombinant) Injection (3 MIU) administered subcutaneously three times weekly.

Patients were treated for 48 weeks and were followed for 24 weeks post-treatment. In the study, patients receiving the 1.0 mcg/kg dose of Peg-Intron achieved a 24-percent treatment response rate of sustained virologic response and ALT (1) normalization as compared to a 12 percent treatment response rate in patients receiving Intron A. (Emphasis added).

**Comment by Lloyd:**

The previous passage, which I have underscored, refers to "sustained response" which means 6-to-12 months non-detected.

The safety and efficacy of Peg-Intron in combination with Ribavirin has not been established.

Nearly all study patients experienced one or more adverse events. The incidence of serious adverse events was similar (about 12 percent) in all treatment groups. The most common adverse events associated with Peg-Intron were "flu-like" symptoms, which occurred in approximately 50 percent of patients; injection site irritation or inflammation, seen in 47 percent of patients; and depression, seen in 29 percent of patients.

WARNING: Alpha interferons, including Peg-Intron, cause or aggravate fatal or life-threatening neuro-psychiatric, autoimmune, isochemic and infectious disorders. Patients should be monitored closely with periodic clinical and laboratory evaluations. Patients with persistently severe or worsening signs or symptoms of these conditions should be withdrawn from therapy. In many but not all cases these disorders resolve after stopping Peg-Intron therapy.

Peg-Intron, recombinant interferon alfa-2b linked to a 12,000 dalton polyethylene glycol (PEG) molecule, is a once-weekly product designed to optimize the balance between antiviral activity and elimination half-life.

Schering-Plough holds an exclusive worldwide license to Peg-Intron. Schering-Plough markets the product as Peg-Intron(TM) in the European Union, where it received marketing approval in May 2000.

Intron A is a recombinant version of naturally occurring alpha interferon, which has been shown to exert both antiviral and immunomodulatory effects. Schering-Plough markets Intron A, the world's largest-selling alpha interferon, for 16 major antiviral and anticancer indications worldwide.

Some 4 million Americans are infected with the hepatitis C virus (HCV) and approximately 70 percent of infected patients go on to develop chronic liver disease, according to the Centers for Disease Control and Prevention (CDC).

Hepatitis C infection contributes to the deaths of an estimated 8,000 to 10,000 Americans each year. This toll is expected to triple by the year 2010 and exceed the number of annual deaths due to AIDS, according to the CDC. The CDC has reported that HCV-associated end-stage liver disease is the most frequent indication for liver transplantation among adults.

Enzon is a biopharmaceutical company developing advanced therapeutics for life-threatening diseases through the application of its proprietary drug delivery and targeting technologies, Peg Modification, Pro Drug/Transport technology and Single-Chain Antigen-Binding protein technology.

Peg-Intron is also in Phase III clinical trials being conducted by Schering-Plough for the treatment of malignant melanoma and chronic myelogenous leukemia. Enzon develops and markets products on its own and through strategic alliances, which in addition to Schering-Plough Corporation include Alexion Pharmaceuticals, Inc., Baxter Healthcare Corporation, Bristol-Myers Squibb Company, Eli Lilly & Company, and Aventis.

Except for the historical information herein, the matters discussed in this news release include forward-looking statements that may involve a number of risks and uncertainties. Actual results may vary significantly based upon a number of factors which are described in the Company's Form 10-K, Form 10-Q's and Form 8-K on file with the SEC, including without limitation, risks in obtaining and maintaining regulatory approval for the Company's products and expanded indications for such products, market acceptance of and continuing demand for Enzon's products and the impact of competitive products and pricing.

The forward-looking statements included in this news release provide the information included in such statements as of the date of this news release and the Company disclaims any duty to update any of such statements.

This release is also available at www.enzon.com.

ALT: alanine aminotransferase, an enzyme that indicates ongoing liver inflammation."

**Article posted to Lloyd's web site message board:**

# SURPRISINGLY LOW IMPACT OF INTERFERON ON HEPATITIS C PATIENTS IN A METROPOLITAN HOSPITAL LIVER CLINIC SETTING

Yngve T. Falck-Ytter, Steedman A. Sarbah, Lucian Sorescu, Kevin D Mullen, and Arthur J McCullough, MetroHealth Medical Center, Cleveland, OH

Background: In the United States, 1.8% of the population has been infected with the hepatitis C virus (HCV) and up to 10,000 die from HCV-related chronic liver disease each year. Current treatment options aimed to eradicate HCV are all interferon based (+/- Ribavirin). In the past, studies have used highly selected patient groups to determine the sustained response rate of interferon therapy. However, the potential impact on viral eradication with interferon therapy in a metropolitan liver clinic's hepatitis C patient population is less well known.

Aims: To determine the proportion of patients who qualify for interferon-based therapy and to identify barriers to treatment.

Methods: All new patients referred to the Liver Clinic from January 1998 to November 1999 were evaluated retrospectively and the reasons for non-treatment and outcome of treatment were documented.

Results: Only 82 patients (25%) of 327 patients evaluated for positive HCV antibody test were started on interferon based anti-viral therapy. Sustained response was achieved in 6 (7.3%), while 12 patients were still in the post-treatment follow up phase. When these data are combined, an estimated maximum of 18 patients (22%) of the 82 patients treated may clear the virus. This would represent only a 6.4% successful viral clearance in all patients evaluated, after excluding patients without viremia (34 patients, 10.4%) and patients currently being worked up (11 patients, 3.4%)). Fifteen patients (18.3%) stopped treatment prematurely because of side effects, 40 (48.8%) were non-responders and 6 (7.3%) relapsed. A total of 200 patients (61.2%) were not treated. Major barriers to treatment included:

1. Seventy patients (35%) had medical contra-indications (depression and other psychiatric disease, decompensated cirrhosis, pregnancy, autoimmune disease etc.);

2. Seventy-one patients (35.5%) were non-compliant with evaluation and education (including incarceration and failure to appear for liver biopsy);

3. Twenty-seven patients (13.5%) had ongoing alcohol and drug use;

4. Twenty-three patients (11.5%) refused treatment with interferon; and

5. Nine patients (4.5%) had normal ALT.

Conclusions: The usefulness of interferon-based treatment of hepatitis C is far more limited than usually assumed. In a typical metropolitan Liver Clinic setting, patients seeking care for hepatitis C will frequently not qualify for interferon-based treatment for a variety of reasons as stated above.

Implications: We hypothesize that focusing on improvement of alcohol intervention and treatment strategies based on decreasing hepatic inflammatory activity may have an even greater long-term impact on morbidity and mortality than current anti-viral therapy.

## Advice for "Newbies"

Hola Lloyd Wright,

I am writing to post my initial test results, recount my experience with the A.M.A. bunch and begin my new path in this life and add to the knowledge base out here for everyone. I think it will be particularly helpful for us "newbie's" to share our stories to help each other make the adjustment mentally and physically to this new crossroads. So bear with me if this initial letter is a bit wordy, it's for the other people that will be following me into these doors to whom every scrap of info might be relevant.

I was diagnosed with hepatitis C in November 2001 after going to a walk-in clinic because of what I took to be a case of food poisoning. I had been in pain for about 4 weeks, and had already self-diagnosed my symptoms as a swollen liver also causing pressure/pain on my spleen. This disruption had all occurred within 30 minutes of having consumed a bean burrito with cheese and guacamole with some M&M's for desert. So I thought that some bad guacamole had produced food poisoning in my liver. I explained all this to the doctor and she felt my abdominal area and checked my posterior for some sort of colonic problem. She then prescribed a liquid for stomach lining irritation (which I tried once and threw away). At least she ordered some blood work done because of my insistence that my pain was in my liver and spleen. While I had been in pain all this time, I instinctively avoided alcohol, fried foods, sugars, junk food, and drank lots of bottled water.

I am already a vegetarian and had given up cigarettes about 7 years ago. My weight is 195 and height is 6'2," so I was already close to having a pretty good lifestyle. Anyway, I tried to keep walking and active because I thought it would help the pain eventually. A few days after the clinic visit, I passed a rather foul-looking blackish stool movement and have felt quite good from then on. I have been a computer contractor for years, so if I am run down, and a in a bit of a fog I always ascribe it to my work, sometimes hellish commutes, and constant moving to follow the jobs. Anyway, I live within walking distance to my job now, which I love, so that part of my life is much better now. I have the love and support of my wife and 4-year-old daughter, and the rest of my family, who give me all the inspiration I need to stay positive and keep everything in perspective.

**Rule # 1, don't freak out.** The clinic didn't call me back, and when I called to get my results, the nurse informed me over the phone of the positive result for hepatitis C, which she assured me was no big deal and she then gave me a referral to a GI specialist. (I had already tried to get an appointment with a GI specialist, but they were all backed up). The doctor at the clinic never called or followed up on me, and I have done all my research online and dealt with all the initial trauma and fears that go with the discovery process by myself. As a computer tech that had worked in major hospitals in the Fort Worth area, I had no illusions the A.M.A. world would have any special concerns for my situation. These hospitals are just very big corporations with insane levels of paperwork, staffed with overworked technical people who are lorded over by administrators and doctors who are produced by hellishly elitist schools to almost completely disregard the observations and concerns of their own nurses and patients.

The GI specialist did the second, more accurate test and I knew enough by now to ask for a full battery to test for other co-infections (I had them check for aids too and I was all clear). Your site Lloyd is just the most helpful in spelling all this out. I can't tell you how much your work means to me and I am sure all the others. I also had my wife get tested, as my biggest fear was that she might have it from being with me. We have a monogamous marriage and have decided that we don't need to use condoms if she's OK now–we've been together about 7 years. She tested negative, which took a huge burden off me.

This new doctor seemed pretty rational and informed at first, and I'll give him big points for making a good effort to allow me time for questions and discussion of this disease.

**Rule # 2, Feel out your doctor's opinion on homeopathic medicine.** Don't let on that you heavily dislike the chemo approach up front.

However, after I felt out my doctor and mentioned that I was doing some research about homeopathic approaches, I got the quick affirmation that his mindset was strictly Peg-Intron with Ribavirin as the only option he would consider valid. Fine, I thought, I need this extra blood work done for now so he can have his opinion. I decided to go ahead with the liver biopsy although I had read about some people's bad experiences with biopsies. I later read your account in your book. Because of you, I knew to make sure that they

223

checked for iron retention at the same time. Last week, I had the biopsy done (deluxe- with local anesthetic) and a "mild" painkiller in the I.V. He had to stick me twice, but no complications from the procedure so far. I definitely think my liver became more inflamed, and I have felt more run-down since then, but I think this will pass with a good homeopathic regimen.

At the end of the biopsy, I agreed to see him in a week to review the results, and he asked me at that point if he should sign me up for the peg interferon & Ribavirin routine, as there is a waiting list. (I guess people are dying to get it yuk yuk–my joke). I told him no, and that I thought I'd wait until our appointment next week and go over my homeopathic research as well as hear his case for chemo in earnest at that point. OK sez he, and I saw signs again of his prejudice against the homeopathic approach but I was determined to give him a fair hearing and also hope for some objective input from him on my research.

I got your book in a devoured it in 2 days–a first rate read and inspiration to all us. Good lord, they can't kill you with a hammer. I think I'm tougher than cheap nails, but if you kept a comin' after all that, I got no problems compared to your scenario. When you feel like you're dying and you know you're pissed, anything less than the truth is an affront of apocalyptic proportions. Thank you for standing up to those leech-hangers and telling the world the truths you've paid for with large pieces of your soul. You can count on me to fight beside you in my own way. (I'm a web-application developer- more on that later).

Anyhow, I go to get my prior full blood work and biopsy results next Wednesday. They told me on the phone before that my blood work had no new surprises, but it turned out that I had been exposed to hepatitis B in the past (that damn burrito?) and I'm supposedly immune to it now, is that so?

**Question:** They said I should get vaccinated for hepatitis A. I've read about this too, do you agree?

**Full Blood work Highlights:**
Flags:
- Phosphorus-    2.2 'low'
- AST (SGOT)-    44 'high'
- ALT (SGPT)-    61 'high'
- Hep. B (S AB)-  150 'high'
- INR            1.1 'low'
- Quantitative PCR Assay, SuperQuant for HCV RNA: "greater than 5,000,000 copies/ml" "equivalent to 2,000,000 IU/ml" (Shit la merde!)
- Hepatitis C Genotype: 1a variant. The sequence of this sample is consistent with minor variations not associated with any subtype.

**Question:** In the above PCR assay, is copies/ml the standard most people in the states use? If so 5,000,000 is the highest I've seen reported so far. My years of stressful work and drinking beer would have been a heavy contributor.

**Everyone**–Don't drink on top of this, I'm proof that alcohol promotes viral replication. I gave up all alcohol upon my diagnosis. My doctor said "you can drink, just don't do it once you are on chemo." Don't believe it!

**Question:** Are there any other items - not flagged, that I should be paying attention to? I can fax you my report if you need it.

**Biopsy Highlights:**
Final Pathological Diagnosis:
- Chronic hepatitis, Clinically hepatitis C
- Moderate to severe activity (grade III-IV)
- Septal Fibrosis (stage 3: this is not good, but it's not catastrophic)
- No abnormal storage iron (good)
- Operative Findings: Grossly normal appearing liver tissue (tan in color)

Microscopic Description:
- Two intact core needle biopsies are examined.
- There is overall preservation of hepatic architecture although distortion is evident centered around the portal tracts.
- There is a moderate to marked inflammatory cell infiltrate, which circumferentially extends into the lobule in most portal areas. This is associated with periportal fibrosis with focal portal bridging, a pattern confirmed by trichrome stain.
- Within the lobule, piecemeal necrosis and Councilman bodies are evident.
- Bile ducts are unremarkable.
- The inflammatory infiltrate consists primarily of lymphocytes with scattered eosinophils and histiocytes.
- Iron stain shows no iron deposition.

**Question:** He said the above II-IV rating was regarding "inflammation". Since 4 is the highest. I presume this is quite bad. What can I do to reduce inflammation? I'm not in pain and don't feel like I've got the "baseball under my ribs" feeling, just a perceived fullness in that area.

**Question:** The Septal Fibrosis looks pretty high to me too, (scale of 4 everybody) what can I do specifically to fight back fibrosis (I'm a 3, isn't level 4 considered outright cirrhosis?)

Well Mr. Wright, Sir, I went to the doktor to get those reports, and have an honest dialogue about options. I made a point of being real courteous and hearing him out first. He reiterated that his only card to play was the Peg Interferon/Ribavirin combo for 12 mos. Oh, and an American Liver Foundation book on how to live with hep C and chemo.

Then asked him about nutrition, as I figured that any doktor would have at least an appreciation of nutrition and liver function. He said that beyond a balanced diet, there was nothing special to do. So I said since the body has fairly complex needs in that arena, I hoped he would refer me to a nutritionist for advice on that only. No dice.

He then launched into his tirade against homeopathic approaches, saying that of the "hundreds" of people he's seen try it, some may have felt better, but no one produced any big results. This is the same man who just told me his practice had only been established for less than a year I think, maybe he was counting his University days. I think he was exaggerating more than a bit. He did mutter something about well, maybe some of the people perhaps just had not reported back to him on their results. He also had no data on what "those people" were using. He said if I have any proof from anyone that "these approaches" work, he'd love to see it. But by his tone I knew anything I told him would be dismissed as unreliable information. Hey– would you like me to send the fool your reports? He also advised me to stay away from Internet message boards! I told him that as an individual with this disease, I considered other people in the same boat to be an extremely valuable and credible source of information. (I delivered that one with all the theatrical understatement I could muster). I also asked him "what if I'm taking the chemo treatment, and during that time, I lose my job and my insurance?" He said, oh, well, there are some programs offered by the drug companies that "might" help. "Like Schering-Plough's "commitment-to-care" program," I asked? "Yes," says he. "I heard you have to be a complete basket case to get that," sez I. He agreed with me. I don't say anymore on that subject, but my research suggests one of the worst things you could do is start chemo then cut it off as your viral load will almost definitely soar. Mine's already high enough.

So, I told him thank you very much, but based upon my own research on the net, and the fact that even his most optimistic data about Peg/Rib accepts a 50% failure rate (higher failure rate for geno 1a's), and the high incidence of damaging, long-term side-effects of chemo, i.e.: higher viral loads, bleeding colon, diabetes 2, etc, that I felt I had nothing to lose by trying a homeopathic regimen first.

Then I asked him if he would arrange for me to come in and have blood work done every 3 months to monitor my progress. He got real peculiar then, and explained to me that "he was extremely uncomfortable doing any lab work for someone not in treatment" (meaning his treatment!) He told me if I insisted, I could come back in 12 mos. He said that every 3 months wasn't practical. So I asked a little later, how often they do blood work if someone is in chemo, and he said 3 months, 6 months, and then 12 mos. I'm not the sharpest tool in the shed, but I know when I'm being "bull----ed." He said, "I don't want to quantify these non-clinical regimens," A little later he said, "Oh, I don't think I don't want to document something new" uh-huh… He danced all around this.

That's why I came up with the rule about not letting on to the doctor about any keen interest in a non-chemo regimen because you might get the bum's rush upfront or even shabbier treatment. I got my initial blood work and the biopsy, so they can kiss my ass. I'll go somewhere else now for follow-up blood work. It would have been a lot of extra stress if I'd had to hop doctors while just trying to get my preliminary stats.

Also for anyone else reading this, not everyone agrees on the need for a liver biopsy. I felt I was strong enough, and my blood is coagulating well. But it's always a crapshoot when you trust anyone to stick a spike into your vital areas.

But my story repeats the pattern that you brought up in your book. The "bas---ds" refuse to keep stats on their own patients, conveniently run off anyone not on their wagon, ridicule any data contrary to their perceived wisdom, and then state with all sanctimony (and a straight face) that no clinical data exists to back up homeopathic regimens. Well "f—k" these fools. I build database-driven web sites for a living and I'm no fool.

Guess what I'm gonna do? I'd like to build a site where us AMA refugees can all go, submit our background information, initial and follow up stats, and the regimens we followed. We'll build our own damn stats and heal ourselves. They can hole up in their ivory towers all day and denounce it, but the bald truth will be hanging out there for all to see. Let me know if you could use my help on your site, or if you'd like to suggest the standardization of information I should try to go with. I may sell advertising on the site someday, but I don't care if I make a nickel on it. I can host it on my home server (1mb bandwidth up & down, cold fusion with sql server backend).

Right now, I'm pretty up on your minimum regimen suggestions, so I'd like to see if you might suggest any specific regimen considering my viral load, stage 3-4 inflammation and stage 3 fibrosis. I am feeling really pretty good. I am a vegetarian, and since about 6 weeks ago, I went all-organic. I am drinking bottled water with a neutral ph, gave up iron frying pans, eliminated hydrogenated oils, eat just a little fried food, cold-pressed safflower oil or extra virgin olive oil. I'm already taking a quality Silymarin extract, 500 mg 3 times per day, vitamin b complex, an herbal detox tea (not milk thistle, the active ingredient eludes me, starts with an 's'), no man-made vitamin A, no nutmeg or sassafras, and walk everyday to and from work, 30-60 minutes a day.

Jesus, this is the most I've typed besides computer code for years. I hope all this detail helps other newbies. Thanks for all your time. I expect to place my first order after hearing back from y'all.

You're a real prince Lloyd. If I can help you with your site, just whistle. I'd be glad to further your message if I can. We'll talk more after this initial load.

Life during wartime,
Bruce Rojas-Rennke
Denver, CO, USA

## Beyond the Medical Hype

Interferon is extremely toxic. For every one person it helps, a score of victims experience its horrific side effects. I do not call this measurable success; I call it a miserable failure. These people are already sick enough with hepatitis C, but because of the FDA and the pharmaceutical companies, they also experience the horrors of interferon treatment, too.

The following nightmarish stories are but a few I have received from people who have undergone much suffering through this supposed "technological marvel."

## Before Peg-Intron, I Was Never Sick

Dear Lloyd,

I just finished four weeks of the Peg-Intron medication and it just about killed me. I suffered all the side effects associated with this. My quality of life went way downhill. I lost ten pounds in the first two weeks.

I hardly slept at all during this time. I was a zombi. I started to become very depressed. I sat in a rocking chair looking out the window all day long. The doctor prescribed Trazodone which made things even worse. My family watched helplessly as I slipped into total despair.

The symptoms did not subside. They became worse. I'm a teacher and with school starting I couldn't imagine myself facing my students. I decided to stop the treatment. It's been ten days, and I'm starting to see my old self again. It's a long struggle back. I'm feeling stronger as the chemicals are flushing out of my system. You know the strange part about all of this is that before I started the "Peg," I was never once sick. The stuff just about killed me!

Back to the herbs!

Peace and Love,
Larry

## They Make It Sound Like A McDonald's Take-Out Meal!

Dear Lloyd,

I've been postponing the new "Peg" combo treatment that my doctor is recommending. One shot a week and Ribavirin pills every day. I don't want to do it. However, my enzymes keep going up, along with my viral load. What should I do? I hear some nasty stuff about this "combo" treatment. They make it sound like a McDonald's take-out meal!

Todd

Dear Todd,

I believe you should avoid the proposed treatment. You could suffer for it the rest of your life. If you are not a genotype 2 or 3a, it is completely worthless, and your doctor probably knows it. Whereas, my program works and you will feel good while doing it.

The prescribing of interferon should be considered a criminal act. It makes the tobacco-industry scandal look like child's play. Pegylated interferon is no more effective than interferon. No published study indicates that interferon works better with Ribavirin than interferon alone. It is a billion-dollar-a-year scam fostered onto sick people.

Lloyd

## I'm Losing My House

Dear Lloyd,

I do not know if you remember me. My name is Mike S. My brother Dan S. told me about you, and we talked on the phone several times. I live in Texas.

Anyway, I did not listen to your advice, and I took the interferon/Ribavirin combo treatment for a year. I thought I was going crazy. My brother sent me your book, but my doctor at Baylor College of Medicine in Houston convinced me that he could cure me.

Well, I had to go on disability for a year, and then I went back to work. My doctor gave me a release saying I was 100% capable of doing my job. Unfortunately, my mind did not function like it should. I would have semi blank-outs and I could not remember people's names, so my company fired me for poor job performance.

Now, after 10 months of being off treatment, I have no insurance and no job. I am losing my house. And, my family thinks I am in a stupor half of the time.

Last month, my "famous doctor" told me that I still have hepatitis C, but the new treatment will knock it out this time for sure. I guess what I'm asking you is: Are there any lawsuits or anything else I can do before I lose my house? If so, could you let me know?

I still have your book but I cannot afford to buy any of the herbs you recommend. I am trying to go on welfare and food stamps. I cannot pay for COBRA. If you can think of any advice, let me know. I should have believed you the first time. I still have $200,000 in life insurance, and I am thinking this might be my only alternative to save my house and get some money for my wife and 10 and 16-year-old children.

Mike S.

Dear Mike,

First, I believe that posting your email to my web site would help many.

Do not use the new Peg-Intron. It does not work! I have talked to hundreds of people who were in the trials. Not one of them is anything but sicker. Peg-Intron is the exact same chemical as interferon except it is time-released. If interferon does not work, Peg-Intron will not work. Your doctor is mistaken!

Peg-Intron was created because the Schering-Plough patent on interferon ran out about a year and a half ago, and they created Peg-Intron to "recapture market share."

My program works and you will feel good doing it. If I were you, I would start taking the following:

> Milk thistle, 400 mg. 3x per day
> Lipoic acid, 200 mg. 3x per day
> Selenium, 400 mcg. 3x per day
> Dandelion root tea, 1 quart per day

These are my minimum recommendation and it can help a lot. Also, take NADH; it really can help with the side effects of interferon. Do it now. Best thing you can do is get your health back, so you can take control of your life. These few items will help, and I can help some.

Lloyd

## Taking Control of Our Lives

Greetings Lloyd,

My husband's hep C diagnosis this past July sent him into a depression that was only made worse by an investigation of the only available "medical" treatment. A subsequent visit to the hepatologist was like entering the twilight zone. This doctor was so accustomed to getting immediate volunteers for his interferon "study" that I think he was genuinely perplexed when we didn't sign on before leaving the office on the first visit.

Our spirits were catapulted by your book! It's only been a few weeks since my husband started with milk thistle and thymus combined with nutritional and immune boosters. The mere existence of an alternative has helped my husband immeasurably. His spirits are higher and his energy is better. This is a path we can follow together, and researching various products and designing a program gives me a way to help him and also gives him the knowledge that he is cared for. We are waiting until November to retest his blood. In the meantime, we can cope and continue with our daily work. This is invaluable.

THANK YOU for your research, for your web site, for your book. You are making it possible for us to take control of our lives and put what the medical world has to offer into perspective.

Ma Kettle

## Last Resort

Hello, Lloyd,

I have just recently bought your book. Is it the only thing that I need to tell me how to get started on getting rid of hepatitis C? About how long will it take if I follow your plan? I have tried the interferon and Ribavirin, which failed miserably, so this is basically my last resort.

Thank you,<br>Donald M.

Dear Donald,

Yes, what is in my book is all you need to do. It requires persistence and some time, but it works and you will feel good doing it.

Lloyd

## Combo Treatment Made Me Extremely Ill

Dear Lloyd,

I am halfway through your book and find it very interesting, but do I need to take all those vitamins? It can be very expensive, as you well know. Which ones do you recommend?

I took interferon with Ribavirin for a year. I became extremely ill (that puts it mildly, I was f----n' sick). I was free from the virus, but it came back after the treatment ended. My doctor wants me to start on pegylated interferon once a week, but I think I will try your therapy first.

Thanks,<br>Bernie E.

Dear Bernie,

Unlike what you get at a good restaurant, the interferon/Ribavirin "combo plate" won't leave you feeling good and certainly won't nourish your sick body. Peg-Intron is the exact same thing as interferon, except that it is time released. My program works and you will feel good doing it. The items in my book are items that your immune system needs to fight the virus. They are nutrients everyone needs, but do not get in their diet. Most of them are not vitamins. Don't do the Peg-Intron. Instead, do at least some of my program. You will be surprised how great it works.

Lloyd

## Ribavirin and Possible Birth Defects

Dear Lloyd,

I am a 39-year-old female with hepatitis C. I was diagnosed in January of 1995. At that time, no real advice on what to do was given to me.

One year later, I saw a gastroenterologist who told me a biopsy was not necessary, and my readings were not high enough to go on treatment. He told me nothing else, so I left it at that.

Then I woke up and decided it was time to do something. I got a liver biopsy. It showed cirrhosis and chronic hepatitis with severe activity and bridging fibrosis, Stage C. Of course the doctors immediately wanted to put me on combination treatment, but I am putting it off for now.

I decided to start your program, but I had to save a little money first. I got most of the products you recommended, except the Natcell Thymus, which I will be getting within the next month. I am altering my diet and starting a mild exercise program.

However, I am still struggling with a few things. I would like to start a family, but I know I have to stay on this program for a while. On the off-chance your program does not eradicate the hepatitis C, I will have to consider the combination therapy.

All of this brings me a couple years down the road, getting older, and making it more difficult to have a child. Sometimes I feel like I should just have the family now and wait to do the program till after that. I know that is really not the right choice, just another item on my plate.

Well, I just wanted to introduce myself, and let you know I am embarking on the program. I will keep you updated. Oh, and thank you so much for your book. It is not only extremely eye-opening, it's witty as well.

Thanks again,<br>Sherie

Dear Sherie,

I know several people who have reversed cirrhosis. I know the doctors do not believe it can be done, but it can.

You need to drink a lot of milk thistle tea and dandelion tea. Also, the Natcell Thymus and Natcell Liver help a lot. Read the Yale School of Medicine article posted on my message board. It clearly states that live cell thymus aids in the regeneration of liver cells. It took years of documenting this success before Yale would ever even look at and acknowledge it.

Keep on doing the program; it works!

Please do not do the combo. It does not work as well as the doctors would like you to believe. If you use Ribavirin, there is a possibility you will not be able to have children because it causes birth defects. Another little something the doctors don't tell you. If you use interferon, you will not want to do anything except die. No joke!

In good health,<br>Lloyd

## High Relapse Rate Of Interferon Users

Dear Lloyd,

I have been on the Ribavirin and interferon for three months, and all my liver enzyme levels are normal. I have Type 1. How long should I expect to be on this medication, and is there any chance of recurrence?

Liver biopsy came back in good condition. They called it a mild exposure.

Best regards,
Clarence


Dear Clarence,

I wish you all the hope and love God can send! The relapse rate of interferon users is high; see my message board for studies. Let me know when you want to get rid of it for good.

Lloyd


## Took Three Shots of Interferon And Quit

Dear Lloyd,

I purchased your book several months ago and inquired about the cost of your treatments. I decided I couldn't afford it. But since then, I've found my symptoms worsening. I was diagnosed with chronic hepatitis C in 1997.

The doctor found that I have cirrhosis of the liver, inflamed gall bladder and spleen. He suggested I take interferon. I took three shots and quit because of the way it affected me.

Now I'm experiencing: no energy, joint pain, severe abdominal discomfort, skin rashes, bloody diarrhea, (and sometimes just blood), and no appetite.

I've decided that right now I really don't have a choice about cost. If you can email me some recommendations as to what might help, I'd appreciate it.

Gene T.

Dear Gene,

I suggest you try following the program outlined in my book. First, considering the symptoms you describe, try properly prepared aloe and Natcell Thymus. If you can't take thymus every other day, then twice a week is better than nothing. Additionally, use the following:

Milk thistle 400 mg 3 times per day
Lipoic acid 200 mg 3 times per day
Selenium 400 mcg per day
Dandelion root tea 1 quart per day
Adrenal 2 a day
Adrenal support is important for liver cell regeneration.
These things will help you.

In good health,<br>Lloyd

## I Don't Want to Mess With the Doctors

Dear Mr. Wright,

I have read your book, and I was very glad for the information. I have chronic hepatitis C, genotype 2 (which the doctor said was a "good" type).

My first viral count back in October of 1999 was 90,000. I know that count was low. I had a liver biopsy the same month, and there was neither evidence of damage to my liver or any cirrhosis.

I did go through the Rebetron/interferon treatment from November of 1999 to April of 2000. At the end of my treatment, I was checked and my viral count was 0.

I went back in November 2000 for another viral check and my count was approximately 260,000 and the doctor said he wanted me to wait (since the count was still low!) until the FDA approved the new pegylated Rebetron treatment, and then do it again.

I waited until May 2001 and took another viral check. My count was up to approximately 360,000. I don't want to mess with the doctor or treatments. I want to do this naturally.

I really appreciate all the hard work and suffering you've had to go through to be able to help your fellow man. Thank you for any help you can give.

Sincerely,
Michael B.

## Another Closed-Minded AMA Robot

Dear Mr. Wright,

I just want to tell you how much I appreciate the fact that you made your story available on the Internet. When my husband was diagnosed with hepatitis C, the first place I went was the net. I know that the AMA has only one objective–to keep their pockets filled while never "curing" anything.

Although my uncle is head of pathology at a hospital and my husband's brother is a doctor, I have learned that the best drugs for the human body are the natural ones.

When the GI doctor talked to us last week, he of course said interferon was the <u>only</u> treatment. I was armed with all the info from the net and asked him about natural herbal treatment. This meek little man turned into a demon who denouncing herbs and the fact that they are "not tested, regulated, or pure," and that he wouldn't give "that stuff" to his own wife.

I politely pointed out that all synthetic drugs pass through the liver and compromise it. He made a few more comments about the "efficacy" of interferon, so I shut my mouth, realizing he was another closed-minded AMA robot.

He wrote in my husband's records: "Wife does not approve of treatment." GOOD! I want them to be aware that I am not going to stand by and watch these V.A. butchers kill my husband!

I am so grateful for all your research and compassion toward others who are suffering from this disease. I am confident that with the information you have provided, and a good naturopath doctor, my husband will be cured. Again, a big thanks!

Sincerely,
Marcia

## Doctor Didn't Really Explain It

Dear Lloyd,

I have the results of my biopsy at last. The doctor says I am level 7, grade 3, and my liver is quite scarred. Do you know what this means? He didn't really explain it, and I was rather confused and upset at the time. Anyway, he wants me to start combined treatment of Ribavirin and pegylated interferon in the summer.

242

I said I needed time to think about it, which he found rather surprising, and I am ordering your book. What is an iron-binding test and why is it important? He didn't say anything about that, only my hemoglobin level.

Oh dear, oh dear, it all sounds deeply depressing. But thanks for your help. I appreciate it.

Claire

## Knowledge is Power

Hello, Lloyd,

I just wanted to say thank you and pass this along. I received a publication from the doctor and it lists the following possible side effects of their combination therapy. I thought you might find this amusing. I am sure it will be interesting reading for others with this disease who are contemplating interferon treatment.

Some of the possible side effects of Rebetron combination therapy, according to my doctor's handout:

> Severe psychiatric adverse events, including depression, psychoses, aggressive behavior, hallucinations, violent behavior (suicidal ideation, suicidal attempts, suicides), and rare instances of homicidal ideation.

I am amazed that you went through what you did and did not kill someone. Knowledge is power. I am so glad that I found your web site. Otherwise, my ignorant self would be taking the poison that can cause the wonderful sensations listed above.

Take care.<br>Randall

## Went Into Clinical Trial Very Positive; After Two Months Discovered It Was Hell

Dear Lloyd,

My name is "Dena." I am 32 yrs old, married, and my husband is virus free. Worked in the dental field for 15 years. I am hepatitis C positive. I gave blood and found out I have this.

My viral load was 200,000 and ALT/AST slightly high. Biopsy shows mild fibrosis. Genotype 1. I tried interferon, Ribavirin and Amantadine on a clinical trial. Went into this with a very positive attitude, only to discover it was total Hell!

I could only do the treatments for about 2 months. Totally freaked out one night. I don't think I could ever try this again. I can't describe how terrible it was.

So now, after 6 months, I take milk thistle (300mg a day). I don't know if this is helping or not. I went back for a blood test to check my viral load on 10-06-2000. It came back 850,000, but my doctor said they changed the way they count it or figure it out now? He said my load is equivalent to 200,000, so I think he means it stayed the same.

Please offer some advice on what I should try except Rebetron. I'm open to any suggestions. Just need help coping with this. My stress level is through the roof. I have 3 young kids. Don't really know where to go from here. Write soon, please.

Thanks,
Dena

## Interferon For 13 Months, Then Virus Came Back

Dear Lloyd Wright!

We just looked up your web site because my sister's condition has recurred. She took interferon alpha 2-b recombinant for 13 months. It held it off for 6 months, then yesterday they said it's come back and she's pretty devastated.

Unfortunately, she lives in a very rural part of Washington, about three hours from Seattle. She can't drive because she's only partly sighted, and she has no medical insurance except Medicare through Social Security (because of her partial blindness).

Aside from the devastation of the treatment not working, she doesn't have much access to people for support groups, etc., and she can't afford a computer so she can go on-line.

So I'm writing in hopes that you'll send her some information. She's very interested in exploring the herbal medicine idea. Thank you so much in advance!

Sincerely,
Scott B.


## Run Through the Mill

Hello, Lloyd,

I just wanted to take a minute and update you as to my situation. I have health insurance which I am sure provided padding for me as I went through the ordeal of obtaining a referral from my Primary Care Physician to see a specialist.

The specialist sent me to the vampire for one of the many blood donations that I have given over the last few months. The specialist ordered a liver biopsy that was a lot of fun when performed on 10/16/00.

I want to know what shape my liver is in and hopefully get accurate information, if that is possible. I already know the next step the specialist is going to recommend, the cure-all wonder drug, interferon.

I like what I read in your book. They can take their interferon and put it where the sun don't shine.

Thanks,
Rafe

## More and More People Cured via Herbs

Hey, Lloyd,

It seems as though I decided to come off drugs at the right time. I keep running into more and more people that have cured themselves of hepatitis C the herbal way. I mean hard-core junkies that must have shot lethal doses of the virus into their veins!

It seems that 9 out of 10 people that take that interferon stuff got miserable from it. The other night at an N.A. (Narcotic's Anonymous) meeting, I met a guy that had hepatitis C and took interferon with absolutely no positive results. He now takes just some herbs, and his counts went down. I know people with HIV and hepatitis C that are doing fine on herbal remedies. I really hope the future holds approvals for the so-called "non-conventional" medicines! Speak to you soon.

Sincerely,
Denny

**Nearly Died From Interferon Combo;
Doctor Told Me To Keep Taking It**

Dear Lloyd,

I have a lot of faith and I believe it is not over for me. I have been taking Aloe Vera, Liver Detox and Milk Thistle because I nearly died from the interferon and Ribavirin treatment.

I actually thought I was going to die before I got better. My doctor told me to keep on taking it. I couldn't climb up the stairs because of weakness. My liver and stomach swelled, and I felt lousy.

He told me the Milk Thistle wasn't proven, and I felt like some kind of clod. I told him my body wasn't agreeing with what he was saying about it. My stomach is still a little swollen, but not as bad, and I don't have any pain.

I am interested in the Natcell and would like more information on it. I lead a natural and active life and this diagnosis has been devastating.

Sincerely,
Alice


**Doctor Going By the Medical Books;
Doesn't Know Anything About the Liver**

Dear Lloyd,

My name is Delores, and my best friend and my sister and I are all hepatitis C positive. We have fought the war of interferon and, to put it mildly, we will not do this again.

I think I have a doctor that is just treating according to what the medical books say. I do not think he knows anything about the liver.

I am trying to find some help for us out there. If you have any information that might be useful to us, please contact me via email or phone me at home. I want to fight a winning battle.

Sincerely,<br>
Delores

## Inter Kill-All

Dear Lloyd,

My name is Bennie B.; I'm the one who ordered a dozen books last week. You called me and we spoke about my brother and sister-in-law, both on "Inter Kill-All."

Anyway, my brother took his last shot a week ago and then called his doctor at John Hopkins in Baltimore, MD. He told him he couldn't take the stuff anymore. My brother and sister-in-law both go for blood work tomorrow to see how the interferon has done. After they get their blood work back, they are going to start on your program, as I have.

Thank you for not giving up on yourself. I love a go-getter. I want you to know I was trying to locate information on a healing clinic when I found you on the Net. Things happen for a reason. God put me in your hands; I know he did. Please keep in touch,

Bennie B.

## Treatment Was Hell And Ruined My Life

Mr. Wright,

I was on treatment for only six months, as was recommended for my genotype. Yes, it was hell and it ruined my life. I still don't know if I am a sustained responder (their term for a successful treatment) because my doctor would not test my viral load (PCR test) until six months after treatment ended, and my insurance had run out by that time.

I will eventually get this test but I am in no hurry, because if the treatment was not successful I would not redo it at this time.

I loaned your book to a few others with hepatitis C, and wanted to thank you for taking the time and effort to share your experience with a fellow treatment sufferer. Again I thank you for your story and thoughtfulness.

Sincerely,<br>Blaine

## After Two Months On Combo Therapy, My Family Thinks I'm Nuts

Dear Lloyd,

My name is "Ruth." I've been on the combination therapy for two months now. All my levels have returned to normal, but the "C" is still detectable.

My family always thought I was a little strange, but now they think I'm nuts. I know it's the medicine, but I'm afraid if I complain too loudly, I will be thought of as a bad candidate for a transplant.

On 9-28-00, I was told I had a 1-inch thrombosis in my left portal vein. Is this reversible? Should I quit now while I still have some sanity left? Or do you think I'm doomed?

I've always been a positive person, but that's been replaced by negativity. Do you have any suggestions? Please reply.

Ruth

Dear Ruth,

My suggestion is that you stop now and use my program. Interferon rarely does more after two months than what it will do in the first two.

If you want to stay on it, I have some suggestions to make it easier. Start taking NADH! Interferon interferes with the neurotransmitters in the brain stem where there are 15 billion brain cells. NADH will help these neurotransmitters work better, and you should feel better.

Also, I suggest that you do as much of my program as possible while you are still on interferon, as it is extremely successful under these conditions. It will help keep you from relapsing, which happens to almost all interferon users (see the article by Dr. Gary Davis on my web site).

Start using the Natcell Thymus and you may become non-detected in as little as one month while on interferon. I have seen this done. I never recommend interferon to anyone, but when someone is already doing it, I recommend several things that can help them survive treatment. The only problem is that these people usually end up giving credit to the interferon. I don't care about the credit, but the facts are the people who have used my program while on interferon are still non-detected. Others I have met in this interferon crusade became non-detected and are now sick again.

I believe that a thrombosis in your vein can be removed. The problem is that many people with hepatitis C die from internal bleeding and many other things that a liver transplant cannot help with.

If you refuse interferon, it cannot be used against you in transplant consideration. If someone told you differently, they are mistaken or lying. It is not in the guidelines that I have. One other thing you can do, which I tried, is cut the interferon dose in half. Doing this did not help me regain my sanity, but it might help you. The doctor thought it would; it didn't.

I chose life over interferon. You must decide which you choose. Regardless, get NADH. It will help and you will need it for a while even if you stop interferon now.

In good health,
Lloyd

## Got The Virus, But Not The Shell

Dear Lloyd,

I was diagnosed 3-4 years ago. Went through the interferon treatments, September-December 2000. We thought we got the virus, but apparently not the shell. The virus has now reactivated. Thanks for your help.

Pat

## Why Do I Get So Nervous After Talking to Doctors?

Dear Lloyd,

I am sending you this info because you said you'd be open to giving me some feedback, which would be most appreciated.

My doctor told me my first viral load count was 187,000 (done in January) and my second (about a month later) was 539,000, with their scale of measure ending at 850,000. She says I am in a state of compensated hepatitis C, (whatever that means).

Why do I get so nervous after talking to these doctors? I said that I had read that these levels were unpredictable, and they were able to be in the millions, and she more or less agreed.

Of course, I want zero counts and am troubled by the fluctuation of almost 400,000 in just a month, though she says it's not that big of a jump. Really? Oh yeah? Easy for her to say!

Ultra sound results: liver, gall bladder, bile ducts, kidneys, pancreas and spleen appear normal. No focal liver lesions or biliary dilation is identified. Mainly she and the liver specialist said everything was very solidly normal, but here's a few ranges I could get out of her:

WBC 4.6, 4.5-11; HCT 41.8, 36-46; PLT 291, 150-350; Iron 129, 30-160; Iron binding 292, 228-428; Liver doctor said ALT is 45 and AST is 42 elevated according to their high normal (in the 30's I think).

He also said albumin, coagulation and a-feto protein normal. He is willing to work with me for a while with my herbal and homeopathic regimen combined with modern German natural pharmaceuticals. I am also using a little machine that pulses current through the bloodstream and claims to remove virus.

FYI: He said there is a new interferon coming out in March-pegylated or something like that, 1 x week and that Ribavirin would not be used. Any poop on that from your "listeners?"

Other than massive depressions from time to time (my life has not been the easiest for the past year—lots of stress on every front) and a troublesome rash on my head, I feel excellent—slightly sensitive in the right liver area, which worsens with stress. Look forward to your input and thanks.

Andrew N.

Dear Andrew,

The numbers you have given me are not bad. It is true that the viral load can change a few million for no understood reason.

Forget the pegylated interferon; it is a lie that it works better. I really need to print a general response letter about this. When the Peg-Intron trials were over several months ago, I had many calls from the sickest group ever.

In good health,<br>Lloyd

## Can You Help?

Dear Lloyd:

Can you help with how much and what should be taken of the alternative herbs, etc.? I have hepatitis C and am taking interferon alpha-2 with Ribavirin. This is my 1st week. My enzymes are normal, but I have an RNA of 93,000.

Dick

Dear Dick,

Stop taking the interferon. It is the worst thing you could possibly do to yourself! My program almost always lowers the viral load by 90% in as little as 30 days, depending on your age, weight, general health, etc. I have had only one non-responder out of several hundred.

The number 93,000 is very low and easy to deal with. If you use interferon, the RNA number will go back up when you stop. People who do it the way I did it stay clear. My best advice is do not use interferon.

In good health,<br>Lloyd

## Interferon Made Me Sicker

Dear Lloyd,

Just thought you might be interested. I wasn't very scientific with all this, but my test results are as follows:

Before:  3/24/2001: AST 97 and ALT 186
After:   5/2/2001: AST 78 and ALT 122

The only thing I did between these two dates was to take frozen thymus for one month. Since then, I have been taking 1,000 MG milk thistle extract daily and one quart of aloe per week.

Prior to 5/2/00, I was on interferon but stopped because it made me sicker (physically and mentally) than not using it. There was also no change in my prior blood results. I think the frozen thymus is an excellent product. In the month that I used it, there was a definite improvement in the way I felt, especially emotionally. I plan on using thymus regularly beginning in June, along with the aloe and milk thistle. Hopefully, this should reduce my results to normal levels.

I'm going to start paying more attention to results, now that I feel there will be some. Thanks again for your book. It has been a great help.

Thank you,
James H.

## No More "Grey Poupon"!

Dear Lloyd,

I just started on the Thymus and herbal remedies recommended in your book. Interferon nearly killed me; I looked as though I had aged 25 years in the 6 weeks I took that vile poison.

Thanks be to God and your program. I now have normal bowel movements, restored energy and optimism, and feel as though my life has been touched by Almighty God and your program in a powerful way. No more dark urine or stools that looks like Grey Poupon!

Thank you, Jesus, for leading me to this 'alternative' remedy miracle!

Janine

## Haven't Touched Interferon

Dear Lloyd,

After reading your book, I began taking Milk Thistle and teas. In two months my ALT dropped from 103 to 44. My AST also dropped from 130 to 76 and I haven't touched any interferon.

Lloyd, your book has been the best inspiration for me. I'm sure I'll be talking to you again soon.

I am impressed, you're THE MAN!

George N.

## Baseball-Under-the-Rib Syndrome
## GONE! –Phone Conversation

This testimony concerns a 56-year-old male who tried the one-year interferon/Ribavirin combo therapy and it failed. His viral load was at 220,000, ALT 166 (1-50), and AST 97 (0-45). He said he'd been extremely sick, fatigued, and nauseous during interferon treatment. He also said that interferon caused feelings of hostility and aggressive behavior, and it caused him to perform acts that were outside his character.

I received a call from his wife only 30 days into my program. She reported that his "baseball under the rib syndrome" (swelling of the liver), which he had been experiencing for several years, was gone.

At six weeks into my program he said, "I feel better than I have in 10 years. I play golf four to five times per week!" A blood test eight weeks later revealed similar numbers as his previous test but he said, "I am not unhappy with the numbers. Even if they stayed the same, I would much rather do this than interferon."

His test dated 6-6-00 indicated that his numbers did eventually drop, his ALT down to 78, his AST to 61, and his viral load at 200,000. His doctor was happy with his improvement and told him that his liver was remodeling.

## Doc Said Only Interferon Would Help

Dear Lloyd,

I was writing to you back in October and you were incredibly helpful and supportive. Besides wanting to thank you, I also want to give you an update.

Since then, my viral load has gone from 3,100,000 to 318,600, down 90% (depending how much one believes in that test). My AST went from 36 to 29 and ALT 61 down to 43. All of this in less than 10 months!

My feeling is that this is because of the thymus, which is the only supplement besides milk thistle that I am diligently taking every day. I could go on and on, but I want to tell you how happy I was to look at the same doctor who told me there was NOTHING I could do besides interferon to lower my counts, and have him read my results now.

Hope all is well with you and I was glad to see your web site up and running well.

Jane

## Another "Spontaneous Remission?"
## Comment by Lloyd:

This client started on my program in August 1999. He had done a year of interferon and the combo therapy, and exhibited anger and hostility beyond his imagination. He indicated that his desire to kill just about anything became an obsession. He reported his intolerance to his doctor who prescribed a tranquilizer and a mood elevator.

He was recently married, and his wife, a registered nurse, stayed with him because she knew that it was the drug causing this bizarre behavior, not the man.

When he started my program, he had been off the interferon for three months. His viral load was 2,200,000. His ALT 215 normal range 0-40 and his AST 210 normal range 1-35.

After three months on my program, he reported that his viral load dropped to less than one million, his ALT was 115 and his AST was 100.

By February of 2000, he reported that his viral load was less than 3.3; hepatitis C non-detected. His ALT was 18 and his AST was 12. This client reported to me that his doctor told him that he "had the luck of experiencing a spontaneous remission."

## No Naturopathic Doctors in This Area

Dear Lloyd,

After my last email, I told you that I had become involved in the Memphis area hep C support group, and that we had never really discussed herbal treatments. Well, I went that night to tell them that we had chosen to stop taking the combo therapy, and they were all very shocked. I told them all about your book and the web site.

The meeting was almost over, and out of nowhere this woman comes marching in the door to tell everyone her great success story on herbal medicines! She also stated that the hardest part about where we live is that there are not any naturopathic doctors in this area. I look forward to hearing from you and pray for your continued good health.

Jean

## Got Hep C While Serving in Desert Storm

Dear Lloyd,

I just wanted to take a minute to introduce myself and thank you for all of the information that you have made available to those of us who truly believed that combination therapy was the only alternative.

First, let me say that I am not infected; rather it is my husband. He is a 38-year-old male, 6 feet, 250 lbs., who has spent most of his life in the gym working out. He's been pretty much the picture of health.

We found out through routine blood work when he had elevated liver enzymes. They decided to run the hepatitis C test, and it was positive. He is totally asymptomatic. The diagnosis was 8/98 and we were referred to a gastroenterologist, known to be the "liver" doctor in our area. He immediately scheduled a liver biopsy to determine the extent of the damage. The biopsy showed chronic hepatitis.

It was determined that he contracted the virus within the past 10 years. Upon taking a extensive medical history, it was speculated that he acquired the virus while serving in Desert Storm through a contaminated batch of gamma globulin in 1991, as the blood plasma products were not screened at that time.

His viral load at that time was over 2 million. The doctor's initial response was to do nothing but wait. Because my husband decided that he had no desire to research the virus, I have made it a mission in my life. At the time of the diagnosis, our two precious little girls were 4 and 1. I could not imagine sitting back and just waiting, so I read and I researched.

He began combo treatment in 10/98. After 48 weeks he was in complete remission. Six months later he was retested and had relapsed. He was told to go back on the combo treatment for 3 months.

That pretty much brings me to where we are today. We just completed the second month of this 3-month treatment, and I called today to tell the doctors that we will not take the third month of treatment.

My husband told me that his one-year of treatment was the worst year of his life, and that he would gladly go back to Desert Storm rather than another year on the treatment.

I have become active in our local hep C support group. It is a fairly small group (normally 15 attend). NO ONE has ever tried any herbal treatments. I would love to have some info from you to take to this meeting. EVERYONE there believes combo treatment and they are told it is the ONLY alternative. One person has had 2 liver transplants, and is currently doing well. One person is currently on the waiting list. One person has had a sustained response from 48-week combo treatment for 18 months; he is our only poster boy for Schering-Plough. Everyone else is either on the treatment, considering the treatment, or waiting!

Stacey

## Another Veteran of Desert Storm

Dear Lloyd,

I was diagnosed with hep C quite by accident during a routine blood test. I am a Desert Storm veteran and have no doubt that somehow the military infected me.

Anyway, I was below 600 in October 2000, and in May 2001 was 1800. Please tell me what SGAT (AST) and SGPT (ALT) means. I am reading the testimonies and would like to know what they mean, and therefore question the V.A. about my counts, which they never gave me concerning those particular letters. Any simple information would be great. Thank you.

Valerie

## Horrible Effects of Interferon Therapy

Dear Mr. Wright,

I read your book on alternatives to the interferon therapy with great enthusiasm. I am now recovering from the horrible effects of trying that therapy, and I want to start your program. How do I go about finding out what dosages of the herbs you used to start with? I'm anxious to get started and look forward to more information from you.

Thank you.
Chris

## Wait Until Bad Enough for Transplant?

Dear Lloyd,

People think I'm an expert on herbal and natural remedies for hep C because I quote from your book all the time. Yesterday I was introduced to a woman named Mary. Her husband was diagnosed with hep C six years ago. He had an allergic reaction to interferon and was taken off treatment. His Blue Cross "doctor" told them that the only alternative was to wait until his liver was bad enough to qualify for a transplant, and he should just suffer in the meantime. This man is only 44 years old and has lost six years of valuable regeneration time!

I gave her your email address as well as your web site info. I hope she follows through. I am calling her tomorrow to convince her to give your program a shot. The "doctor" has advised her husband against natural remedies, so she needs enough information to convince him. Thanks again for your help, you'll be getting an order from us soon!

Roxanne

## Daughter Worse After Interferon

Dear Lloyd,

Our daughter is very bad. She took interferon, and her test results following treatment showed no improvement. Instead, she was worse. She is now starting that treatment over again, along with some by-mouth medication. Doctors tell her that if this doesn't help, nothing is left except possibly alternative medicine.

Thank you in advance for answering this email and any other comments you would care to make.

Alice

## Pressured to Get on Interferon Study

Dear Lloyd.

I was diagnosed with hep C three years ago. I feel okay. Liver enzymes normal. Every time I see my hep MD, he pressures me to get on studies, including interferon, etc. My genotype is 2a.

My husband died on 10/28/99 after his second liver transplant due to hep C. He took interferon for years, and it made everything worse.

I've been using milk thistle and reishi mushrooms occasionally. I am very interested in the alternative route! Any info will be very much appreciated.

Thank you,
Gail

## Interferon is a Liquid Nightmare

Lloyd,

Thanks for your timely response. I'm a bit overwhelmed recently, especially with my doctor ready to inject me with this liquid nightmare (interferon). It just appears to me, especially from the onset, that there is very little a person can do about this "chronic" condition. Conventional medical wisdom is really pushing this "combo" on me. I've been putting it off for 5 years.

I'm 32 years of age. Sometimes I wonder if I'll be around to see my daughter graduate high school. Anyway, I don't mean to depress you. I really need to get a handle on this stuff instead of pushing it to the back burner.

Todd

Dear Todd,

It may be that the smartest thing you have ever done is to make the decision NOT to take interferon. Many have permanent damage from it. It has a very low success rate, less than 1% over 3 years, a terrible waste of life.

If you want to get well, read *Triumph Over Hepatitis C* and follow what it says. I have a 97% success rate with those who use the program as directed. It is a little expensive. I mortgaged my house, rented it out, and moved into a barn to pay for it. I figured I had two choices, die or maybe live and be broke. I never expected to be saving thousands of lives. It works on just about everyone.

Just get started! I have several people on my program who were patients of a particular doctor. Many of these people were on all sorts of strange medical programs. Some were taking 10,000,000 units of interferon a day for a year. They are sicker now than they ever were.

In good health,
Lloyd

## Heartbroken and Depressed

Dear Lloyd,

My dear brother John is 44 years old and has hepatitis C. He is currently on interferon treatments. His 5-month checkup is next week. He sees a doctor at Yale New Haven hospital.

I am heartbroken and devastatingly depressed by his misfortune. How can I encourage him to consider an alternate route in his therapy? We don't want to lose him.

Sincerely,
Mary Ellen

Dear Mary Ellen,

Hopefully, he has suffered enough. If the interferon has cleared the virus, he should read the volumes of info that state clearly that it comes back. Several pages and studies can be found on my site.

When one is on interferon, the immune system goes to sleep. The virus is very small and sometimes becomes undetected because the tests are not good enough to detect it (see the article by Dr. Gary Davis on my web site).

Then, while the immune system is asleep, the virus begins to re-grow. This is the optimum time to start my program. It helps build the immune system and kill the virus. Even if the virus is not non-detected, it may have mutated to preserve itself against interferon and it is time to get it.

In good health,<br>Lloyd

## Don't Know If We Should Try the Drugs

Dear Lloyd,

My husband tested positive 4 years ago for hep C. On December 4, we are seeing the doctor who will be giving him prescription for interferon (I think). It entails one injection a week and 5 pills a day.

I am very worried. He's very thin to begin with. On November 12th, he had his liver biopsy. All the doctor told me was it is stage 1 (mild). My husband is 37 years old and we have 2 small children.

I am getting even more worried now. I don't know if we should try the drugs the doctor recommends. I spoke with a nurse who works for the pharmaceutical company and she said no vitamins, especially no iron.

I just wanted to let you know my situation, and I plan on doing more research.

Smiley

Dear Smiley,

Please do not let him use interferon. He will never be the same. Even if it works, the virus will come back. Have you read everything about Peg-Intron on both my web site and the CDC web site? The stuff should be considered criminal. He is too young for this. I have seen too many people ruined by this poison. Blindness, neuro-psychiatric disorders, autoimmune disease, thyroid cancer, kidney failure, etc. I really hate seeing this happen.

Most of the people I have communicated with, who have done the interferon/Peg-Intron treatment, have never been the same. They have viral loads 3 times higher than before. The doctors are making money on this, and neither the doctors nor their patients know about anything else.

Please, read everything you can before doing this destructive cancer treatment for a virus. Many people who use my program get well; almost all of them return to normal life. If you answered my phone for even one day, you would never consider interferon.

In good health,<br>Lloyd

## By-passing Interferon

Dear Lloyd,

I would like to know if any one has tried your program without ever having tried interferon. If so, what were the results? This is important to me. I have unknowingly

265

passed hep C to my son. I would like to spare him the treatments.

Carl

Dear Carl,

A year ago I could tell you I followed 32 people who were on the program with success. Today, I can tell you there are so many that I cannot keep track. I am so overwhelmed that I don't have time to eat. So I will guess, a few hundred.

Lloyd

## All Your Work May Save My Life Now

Lloyd,

I read your book and did more research on HCV. I pretty much had my mind made up to take the herbs, but wanted to speak with my doctor to see if any of them would affect my high blood pressure.

I know you hate the doctors, but I have a good one Lloyd. After we took all of the regular stuff, I told him that I wanted to talk to him and that I wasn't looking for his approval, but for his cooperation. I had your book with me. I told him what you had advised me to take. He was very interested in knowing what each item could do for me. I had the book marked, and opened it to each page as we talked of each item. He has no problems with anything. He said that he even takes selenium and thinks it's great.

We did talk about the new pegylated interferon that is supposed to come out after the first of the year. The only thing he asked me to do was that if the herbs do not help, would I then consider the new interferon. I was honest with him and said I would consider it, but I would not promise. He was fine with it all.

I explained a little about your situation, and told him that you are not a doctor, but a patient who was intent on living. He took your book from my hand and wrote your name and your web site down. I think he will take a good look. He has an open mind about the whole thing.

I am on a mission and I have a goal. I thank you to the bottom of my heart for the hope and assistance you have given me. I will let you know how it goes. All the work you did may just save my life now.

Thank you my friend,<br>Nancy

Dear Nancy,

I have many people on my program who have done the pegylated interferon trials. These people all say they are sicker than when they started. They are the sickest in terms of disability that I have experienced.

Pegylated interferon chemically is not different than normal interferon except that it is time-released. Doctors are really pushing it, and the drug companies are really plugging it as being effective. Doctors all across the country are thinking it is great, and I think some of this is the BS from the drug companies, and some of it is because of money. The reality is that the trials, which have been going on for at least two years, have not had the success that is being put out there.

It does, however, cause a temporary jump in stock prices. And that is not a joke.

Lloyd

## Doc Recognizes Interferon Failure

Greetings, Lloyd,

Beginning in about September, my husband began a supplement program using many of your recommended supplements, including the live cell thymus. He's predominately stage one with movement toward stage two, and his numbers are around one million.

The first MD was an interferon pusher, and we backed off and followed your advice instead. The second MD (the lead man in Miami at the University hospital) was a real human being. His advice: continue with the supplements, see him twice a year, and wait until a better alternative becomes available. He runs a variety of trials and has been recently approached with funding for a trial using many of the same supplements my husband takes, except they are taken intravenously. So, he was sympathetic and non-judgmental. This latest "natural" trial is being targeted for hep C's who have already tried interferon, so we're not eligible.

My point is, my husband continues to take your advice and, though we haven't retested him yet, he feels better just by having an alternative that allows him to take active part in his health care. Also, we are relieved to have found an MD who has enough knowledge to understand that my husband's hep C does not require a rush to use drugs that don't work, and who won't discuss the potential of natural supplements.

So we are "hanging in there," and feeling grateful for the work you do that allows us to be active in our fight against hep C.

Thanks,
Mary Anna

Dear Mary Anna,

Who is your doctor? I would like to know. Also, I would like to post your email on my message board if it is all right with you. I like the letters that relate a story about a doctor who recognizes the failure of interferon and combo. Please let me know.

Happy New Year,
Lloyd

## Progress News!

Dear Lloyd,

My husband has been on your program since February of this year. I just wanted to let you know that he is doing great. His liver counts are in the normal range (which they have not been since 1996 when he first diagnosed with hepatitis C!). His viral count is at 850,000, which is down also. He feels the best he has felt in years. We actually lead a normal, active life now.

Before we found your program on the Internet, my husband went through the interferon combo treatment. What a nightmare! Never again. He felt worse than ever before and could barely function. His only activity was to make it through the work day! Now that he's on your program, life is so much better. I have faith that this will cure him in time. It's amazing the peace of mind that I have had since starting my husband on your program. It's just a part of our lives now, and I can focus on other things in life instead of spending literally hours searching for something that would cure (or even help) him, since conventional medicine does not appear to be doing anything about finding a cure for hep C.

I can't thank you enough for sharing your information and experiences. You have given hope to people dealing with hep C. I just hope that anyone living with hep C (whether they have it themselves or just live with someone who has it) takes advantage of your program and information. You've accomplished what the medical industry has not in dealing with hepatitis C.

I also commend you on your web site and ordering process. It is so user-friendly. There is a wealth of information on the site. The ordering procedure is easy to follow and the secure site for entering a credit card number makes me feel comfortable ordering "on-line."

We have placed several orders with you and have never had a problem. We have always received what we ordered in a very timely manner. What great service. I have to admit that at first my husband and I were a little skeptical of your program only because we had found other web sites that just didn't sound sincere. But after ordering your book and reading it, we both agreed that no one could write about the experiences you had and have the knowledge you did unless you actually went through them.

We could relate with you throughout your entire book because we, too, have been there! We also felt that anyone who had gone through the experiences of dealing with hep C could not, in good conscience, take advantage of others. Personally, after reading your book I was so excited about it that I couldn't wait to get started! The best thing we did was to purchase your book!

Most of all, I would like you to know how impressed I am with you and your obvious willingness to help others. You have always answered my emails within 24 hours (and that's only because of the time difference; otherwise, I am sure it would be sooner). No question or concern is too trivial. You are truly a remarkable person.

I hope you post this on your message board so that others can read it. I hope it gives faith to those already on your program and I hope that it encourages others to try your program because, believe me, it really gives you peace of mind to know that you're doing something to help yourself or a loved one fight against hepatitis C.

People need to know that they're not alone in dealing with this, nor is the situation totally hopeless!

I'll keep in touch! Have a great day and God bless,

CD

## Human Guinea Pig?–Comment from Lloyd:

Everyday I hear stories from victims of hepatitis C that would be easily dismissed as fiction by the medical community, not to mention the average American.

With their arrogant attitudes and demeaning behavior, many doctors just smile and chuckle when asked about the healing potential of herbs. However, some of the success stories I've heard from my clients can't be dismissed with a chuckle and a smile. In fact, a good number of their stories even out-do my own personal account.

For example, today I heard from a client of mine from Arizona. She's forty-two years old and only three months ago underwent gallbladder surgery. She had a liver biopsy performed during the procedure. The results of the biopsy were clear: chronic hepatitis C, stage 2 cirrhosis. The hepatologist told the patient her condition was too bad to treat with interferon and that she would need a liver transplant, and he put her on the transplant list.

After some research, the woman read my book, *Triumph Over Hepatitis C.* She liked what she saw, and she decided to give the program a try. After three months of the program, she returned to see the doctor at the University of Arizona Teaching Hospital. Upon seeing her, the doctor admits he did not expect to see her looking so healthy.

She told the doctor that she has been taking herbs. Immediately the doctor stated, "I must have been wrong, I must have made a mistake when reading your reports." The lady retorted "listen to me, I've been taking herbs."

Ignoring her, the doctor handed her a form to sign so he can acquire the slides of her biopsy to reexamine them. Then he said, "You can not get well from this condition."

I would love to meet this "fool" in a public forum and debate him on these issues.

Another terrific story unfolded recently. Three weeks ago, a forty year-old female called me. She sounded near death, weak, confused, hopeless, and definitely much older than her age. She told me that following my program cured her friend. She told me that she has read my book and that she needs help because her doctor is killing her. She enlightened me on the horrors she has faced. She says her doctor has had her on interferon since 1997 (11 months on, 2 months off, 11 months on, 2 months off for four years). I told her that she should already be dead. She then said that she has been on pegylated interferon for 5 weeks.

We talked for a couple more hours, and the whole time she's telling me how terrible her life has become. Her husband was on the phone for some of the conversation and he confirmed her troubles.

She then told me she has had four liver biopsies. When she read them to me, I'm thought to myself, "these are the best liver biopsies I've ever heard." She then stated that her doctor told her that her viral load was off the charts, that it was so high it couldn't be measured.

The test she was given was PCR RNA HCV Qualitative, the test with a range that just stated, "greater than 850,000."

I thought this is beginning to sound like she was used as a guinea pig to determine the long-term effects of interferon. I know that not many people could tolerate interferon for that length of time. She was the perfect victim because of the simple fact that she kept on being a victim.

Then she told me she had pleaded with the doctor to let her stop the pegylated interferon, but he stated that she would die if she stopped.

I pleaded with her and her husband to stop the insidious criminal activity being perpetuated by the doctor. She obliged and stopped taking interferon. She went on my full program. After a few days, her husband called me late at night. He asked me, "What have you done to my wife?" He told me that when he came home from work he found the house clean, cleaner than it had been since his wife had begun taking interferon. He said his wife had also taken down and washed all the curtains. He happily told me that he and his wife spent the rest of the evening putting the curtains back up. He had his wife back, and I could feel his joy through the telephone.

These are just two of the success stories I've heard recently. If I wanted to document everyone I've heard about I would have to take off a couple years to do it, so for now, I will keep you keep sending along a few stories of hope as I have time.

How long will it take before "doctors" realize that the health of their patients is more important than the money that finds its way into their overstuffed wallets? Hopefully, not too long.

## Peg-Intron–Comment from Lloyd:

During the last several months while this book has been under construction, numerous stories have poured in about Peg-Intron. None of them have been anything short of unbelievable disaster. I need to relate this one, as it is one of my favorites.

Three New York Prison guards were diagnosed with chronic hepatitis C. Two went on Peg-Intron and one went on my program. All three have the same doctor.

In one week, one of the Peg-Intron victims was incarcerated for repeated suicide attempts; the other was disabled and prescribed several tranquilizers, mood elevators, and pain medication.

The prison guard that is on my program is still working, and his viral load is dropping 100.000 to 150.000 a month.

The insurance company for the prison guards decided to pay for my program because it is far cheaper than disabling workers with Peg-Intron.

Peg-Intron is not what the drug companies what us to believe.

## A good day on the peg was a day he could lift his head off the pillow–Comment by Lloyd:

Just one more testimonial that came to me yesterday:

A 52-year-old male called me yesterday and then faxed me his blood work because his doctor did not have time to explain it.

He was on my program for two months when his doctor convinced him to try Peg-Intron for a study being offered.

When he stopped my program and started Peg-Intron, his viral load was 1.904.149. That was on 11/29/00. Six months of Peg-Intron and his viral load was 4.455.710.

He told me that a good day on the peg was a day he could lift his head off the pillow! That is an exact quote.

He started back on my program, realizing he had to live with this and interferons are not life-friendly.

On 9/18/01 his viral load was 3.570.492. His next test was on 1/9/02. His viral load was 2.160.289. His SGOT 32, his SGPT 35, Protein, total, serum 7.2, Bilirubin, Total 0.5.

The rest of his blood work is also perfect with the exception of WBC count, RBC count and Platelet count being on the low side as a direct result of the negative effects of Peg-Intron.

## The Dr. FINALLY Took Him Off of It

Dear Lloyd,

Thanks for the information that you sent. As of a couple weeks ago, Harry became so ill taking that new medication, Peg-Intron, with a severe rash at the injection site, and just always sick, so the Dr. FINALLY took him off of it.

It was but a month later and Harry developed Type 2 Diabetes. After his hep Dr. called the company, it was found that several of the people taking Peg-Intron and the other medicine had also gotten Diabetes. However, it cannot be proven that it came from this drug, even though it seems that is the likely cause. But because Harry agreed to take the medicine, it is most unfortunate for us, because if I could I would slap someone with a law suite, even though it is not listed as a side effect.

So we are back on the Herbal Meds. And I have my ol' Harry back again.

Sincerely<br>Kathy

## So Much For That Theory

Dear Mr. Wright,

I just finished your book *Triumph Over Hepatitis C*, and I found it very informative. I tested positive for hep C 2 years ago. Last year I went through 6 months of interferon combo treatment. I had cleared it at the end. Then last week after my 3-month follow-up test, I learned that it had returned. I just got back from the doctor's office where he told me I had 3 choices: Peg-Intron (a new protocol of interferon). He said I would have to go on small doses for the rest of my life. Since I am only 39 years old, this did not sound appealing, so I talked about thymus and milk thistle. He comment was it wouldn't help, but it could not hurt me. He told me to come back in 6 months to retest. I would like to give your program a try, but you have so many products. I am not sure which to order and I do not have unlimited funds, but I want to get the best program I can so I can have good results. I am also unsure of the proper dosage. I am a 39-year-old male. I weigh 260 lbs. I life weights 5 days a week and also 5 days of cardio workout. My body fat is 11% and I am 6'4". I follow a fairly good diet, but after reading your book I'm not so sure! I like red meat and aspartame. So any help you can give me would be appreciated.

I would like to get started a.s.a.p. Also I have type 3-a hep C, which is supposed to be the easy one to clear on interferon. So much for that theory! My AST today was 45 and my ALT was 99. They did not do a HCV count, only a test to see if it was positive.

Thanks,<br>Brad Larson

## I love red meat too.

Dear Brad.

I love red meat too, but would like to let people know that they need to shop wisely. Where I live they have organic, grain-feed beef. I suggest that you use sugar instead of artificial sweeteners, forget the negatives you have heard about sugar. I've read that aspartame is a very dangerous neuro-toxin that can cause seizures, even in folks without epilepsy. If interferon did not work, which it does not, Peg Intron will not. They are the exact same molecule, only time released.

I suggest you take the following supplements:

Milk thistle 400 mg 3 times per day
Lipoic acid 200 mg 3 times per day
Selenium 400 mcg per day
Dandelion root tea 1 quart per day
Then if you can afford more
Natcell Thymus 1 vial every other day
Aloe 4 oz 3 or more times a day, and
the rest of the things in my book.

Your doctor is wrong! I will send you a copy of my new book for you to look over. Read it and tell your doctor he should open his eyes and read it too.

Lloyd

# SEVEN

# HEALING TEAS

I call this my "just for fun" chapter. I love it when clients really get creative with mixing the teas and herbs to suit their own individual tastes. I almost expect to see one of them become the "Julia Child of Herbal Detox" one of these days.

Occasionally, I get a letter from someone who will ask, "What are these weird teas?" Well, a good description of the teas, and the herbs from which they are derived, is given in my first book, *Triumph Over Hepatitis C.* Even though many of these teas and herbs are foreign to our current junk-food diet and mentality, they have been used to help people maintain good health for thousands of years. They actually can become quite tasty with a little practice.

As you can see from the sample letters below, my clients have learned to embrace the flavor of the teas that heretofore may have tasted "weird" to them. See what a little creativity can do? One person even coined a new word to me: "Vege-quarian."

## Can Hear Hope In Dad's Voice Again!

Dear Lloyd,

The dandelion tea is so far a success. I got my dad some of it early this week and he called me last night and said it was working. He said he was able to get out of bed and eat, and he also went out into the yard. This made me so happy. I can't thank you enough.

I know we have a lot more to do, but it's a start. He had given up, but now I can hear hope in his voice again.

From,<br>
Tim

## Licorice Tea Recipe and Feeling Great!

Dear Lloyd!

I made the licorice tea, and it turned out delicious! I made a drink of sorts. I take two ounces of the aloe vera juice, one ounce of lemon juice, and mix it with the licorice tea. Then add ice, and it's a delicious drink! I don't use artificial sweetener or sugar, but it tastes delicious anyway!

Well, I am feeling great! I have more energy than I have had in a long time. My mood is better than ever. I had been so blah and so depressed for so long that I forgot what it was like to feel "normal," whatever that is!

Lately, I go to work and get so much done! I seem to just glide through work. I used to hate getting up in the morning. It was a chore just getting out of bed. I wanted to sleep all day. Once I got to work, I would feel so sick all the time. I would be nauseous, fatigued, depressed, and I would have a headache that never went away.

I felt like the end of the day was never happening quick enough. Does all of this sound familiar?

I can only imagine at this point what you must have felt like. If this good feeling I have gets better, plus if I get well on top of it... wow!

In the beginning of all of this, when a person with hep C starts taking the Natcell Thymus, all the supplements, etc., is the body going through a kind of "detoxing" period? It just makes sense to me that it does.

So, are all of these things we take in the beginning fighting the virus? Is there a kind of war going on inside the body? If so, wouldn't there be a kind of storm before the calm? Don't we kind of feel these changes as we detox from all the poisons the hep C virus caused and don't we feel the changes while the virus is being stirred-up?

So, as usual, I thank you so much! Also, if you need to, you can always put my emails and your responses to them on the message board if it would help others.

Robert

## "Vege-quarian" Keeps HCV at Bay

Dear Lloyd,

I think that what has kept my hepatitis at bay for so long is the fact that I have been a "vege-quarian" for the past 8 years (fish two or three times a week), and I have been taking a lot of antioxidants and colloidal minerals. I had acupuncture today and feel great. I'm brewing some bulk milk thistle right now. I drink only distilled water. I'm simmering 1/4 cup of the herb with 2 quarts of distilled water for two hours. I also enjoy the reishi mushrooms twice a day.

Thanks for returning my email. It really means a lot to my wife and me. Thank you again, Lloyd!

Doug

## Craving Olives Lately

Dear Lloyd,

Got the book and couldn't put it down. Just finished and placed a small order for some items. I was interested in the olive leaf. I have had cravings for olives lately and, though a life-long olive hater, I now have an olive sandwich a day because it tastes so good. Coincidence, who knows. I also find my general diet tastes have changed toward much less meat and more raw veggies. I crave the sunshine, which is a real problem here on Misery Point, so close to the Olympic rain forest. Anyway, I think we can learn from our bodies if we can stay out of old habits and keep an open mind.

On a less sanguine note, my first friend died of hep C. I got the news today. Oh boy. Let's live well you and I. Consider a vacation in Thailand; it makes life very worth living.

Adios for now,
Dennis

## Something's Working

Lloyd,

I had my first experience with simmering in glass. My wife wasn't here to direct me, and I shattered the Pyrex and had reishi in, on, and under the stove!

Your book says simmer 8 cups of water with 20 slices of reishi and then dilute by 50%. Am I correct?

Thanks for all of your continued support. Incidentally, my ankles are no longer swelling and my chicken legs are back. Something's working.

Bill

## Struggling To Keep Grin Off My Face

Dear Lloyd,

Thanks for the info. I'd be definitely interested in the powdered milk thistle and beet leaves.

The thymus was a bit of a surprise. I was wandering around feeling very tall and struggling to keep the grin off my face. I thought someone might have slipped something into my scrambled eggs.

I haven't got any great recipes yet, except to say that a lemon squeezed into the top of a glass of cat's claw tea confuses the taste buds long enough to get the horrible stuff down.

Regards,<br>
Brett

## Dressing Up Tea!

Lloyd,

Thank you for the reply. I'm so excited about this program I didn't want to risk having my supply of thymus cut off.

I'm trying to step up the tea part of the program. Yuck! I've managed to dress up some of your recipes and thought you might like to share this info with others. I add the juice of 1 - 2 lemons to each batch of dandelion and cat's claw. I also pick a few mint leaves from my garden and add to the batch when I'm ready to refrigerate. It helps tone down some of the bitterness. Don't add these ingredients to the licorice root as it clouds up and looks like it's spoiled.

Thanx,<br>
R.

## Seems Like A Lot of Tea

Lloyd,

First I want to thank you for your book. I admire your courage and tenacity in finding something that worked for you. I also want you to know how much I appreciate that you are so willing to spend as much time, as you must, to email and answer everyone's questions. I have to imagine that is overwhelming at times.

My husband was diagnosed with hep C a couple of years ago. He contracted it in a very similar way to the manner you did. He had a JD tractor roll over on him when he was 12. He suffered severe injuries and had many blood transfusions.

Anyway, we have run into similar experiences with the medical industry. We sort of decided that there was nothing we could do. He was feeling pretty good at the time. Things aren't so good anymore. I've been doing some research on my own. I came across your web site and have investigated what I can about your recommendations. I'm very impressed with what you've done. I'm also impressed that you seem to have made the products available at a cost that is much lower than I can find elsewhere. I want to thank you for that!

I have several questions: Why is it important, or is it, to make the various teas while taking the same thing via capsule, etc.? (Seems like a lot of tea.) If we start on the Natcell Thymus, should we order what we need for a month at a time or what do you recommend?

Our regular family doctor is willing to run blood tests on a regular basis for us. The hepatologist is not thrilled that we are rejecting the interferon treatment that he recommends. He also isn't thrilled and doesn't want to know about alternative treatment. Should we be looking for a doctor that does deal with herbs and supplements, or go it on our own? Thanks for all you do.

Bless you,
Joy

Dear Joy,

The teas have things in them that are not in the processed capsule. They are very important. Most people do not like them. But they are necessary, at least milk thistle and dandelion and hyssop. I suggest ordering as much of the Natcell as possible to cut down on shipping cost. That is what I did.

The hepatologist sounds like a normal hepatologist. It is very hard to find a good naturopath or nutritionist. They all have their own ideas, or they are undereducated about live cell protein. Most of the people who try to find themselves a naturopath or nutritionist end up spending a lot of money on them. That is up to you. Most just try and do the program on their own–with help from me.

Lloyd

## Your Teas are First Rate!

Dear Lloyd,

I'd like to make sure I'm following your program correctly, and I have a couple of questions. Before I get into that, I would like to tell you how pleased I am with the teas. They are simply first rate! There's simply no comparison between your product line and what I was getting in the health food stores. They are just fantastic.

I'll give you some more feedback. I started with the Natcell Thymus and Liver and most of the herbs. However, I still have not received the Aloe or Eurocel. I realize it has only been six days, but I must admit I already feel better. I'm still tired, but my mind sharpened right up, and I'm very pleased about that. As you suggested, I now have a copy of every test that was completed on me. There are a lot of them, but the main ones read:

HVA Viral Load greater than 850,000 IU/L, AST 47 IU/L, ALT 59 IU/L, Genotype 1a; ultrasound of liver normal. I will have these tests again in three months so we can see if any modifications should be made to my treatment.

I have two questions. When we talked on the phone, I thought you said I should take 7,000 mg. of Vitamin C three times per day to tolerance (which I am able to do without a problem). However, in your book it says you took 7,000 mg two times per day for three months and then you dropped it to 2,000 mg two times a day. What do you recommend? Also, in the book you say you took 500 mg of dandelion root three times per day. However, I did not get it in my three-month supply. Was that an oversight, or do you think the tea is enough? If I need the capsules, I'll get them. Let me know what you think.

Thanks for your help,

Bob


Hi Bob,

I sent your Eurocel a few days later because I ran out. You should have it in a day or so. If not, please let me know. I think I sent it FedEx.

I'm so happy you like the tea. I have so many people buying it from the health food stores, and I know what I provide is a lot different. I would like to post that part of your message so people can get an independent idea for themselves.

The aloe takes a week to 10 days to arrive. It weight 20 pounds per box, and it is expensive to ship, so it goes Fed Ex Ground.

My recommendation is that you take vitamin C to tolerance, meaning you should take as much as possible without causing problems such as diarrhea. I now have a liquid vitamin C derived from beets in 10 gram bottles (equal to 100,000 mg.) Because of the way it is made, it is nearly as absorbable as injections and does not have negative side effects. Dandelion root tea is much better than taking the capsules. I only carry capsules for people who will not drink the tea and for others when they are traveling and cannot make the tea.

The viral load test you have is a range test. It simply says greater than 850,000. That could mean 851,000 or 100,000,000. It would be nice to have a test with an exact number so you can see how fast it drops.

When you have further questions, I am here.

Lloyd

## Nothing Short of Miraculous

Dear Lloyd,

I'd like to give you some feedback about my reaction to your program. So far it's been nothing short of miraculous. On 9/25/01 I was diagnosed with HCV. I had been feeling a little off for a couple years but couldn't but my finger on the problem. Previously I hadn't been to a doctor for over 25 years. I always felt great, until now. After returning from a vacation that involved heavy drinking, I felt terrible. I had a feeling it was more than just a hangover. I scheduled a doctor's appointment and had numerous blood tests, and that's how I found out. The doctor scheduled an ultrasound and referred me to a doctor of hepatology. I went home, got on the web, and started studying the disease. I was shocked and scared. After the ultrasound, I went to the liver specialist who suggested a biopsy and then Rebetron combo therapy. I told him I wanted to try modification of my diet and the herb therapy I was

287

reading about on the web, but he was not impressed. He ordered a genotype test and set a follow-up appointment. It was time for me to make some important decisions. My health situation was severely affecting the quality of my life. I was tired. I had to nap 2 to 3 times a day. I could feel my liver almost like heartburn all the time. I had terrible memory problems and difficulty concentrating. At this point, I was reading every book I could get my hands on and spending hours on the web gathering information and perspectives. The list of side effects associated with interferon scared me, and I was hoping to find a different, more credible course of action. I changed my diet to nothing but organic foods, no caffeine, no alcohol, no aspirin, and I bought a vegetable juicer and organic cookbooks. My theory is that I'll only put things in my body that are good for my liver and immune system and nothing else, in order to give my liver a chance to rest and regenerate. I've always worked out, but I've become more serious, 5 days a week, even if I'm tired. I bought the herbs I read about and started taking them. After about 10 days, I felt better. One of the books I read was yours. I got on your web site and was intrigued that you had cleared the virus. I called you against the advice of my mother, who is a nurse, and my doctor, who wants me to start interferon/Ribavirin therapy. We spoke on the phone, and because I was encouraged by your enthusiasm, and my fear of the side effects of interferon, I decided to try your program for the 18-month interval. I ordered a three-month supply including Natcell Thymus and Natcell Liver, which is expensive. However, I have no prescription drug coverage with my health insurance and surmised after consultation with my doctor that your program is about the same price as combo therapy. Combine that with the fact that if it worked it would be abundantly less expensive because I could keep working through the treatment. I received my Natcell order 10/24/01 and most of the rest 10/26/01. With my diet modifications and herbal supplementation I felt better, but my health situation was still severely affecting the quality of my life. I started your program 10/24/01 and felt better every single day. For the last year and a half the lymph glands on the sides of my neck have been swollen like walnuts. On the eighth day after beginning your program, when I woke up in the morning, the swelling was GONE! I am stunned, I feel better than I have in two years after only EIGHT DAYS! My memory's back; I have no difficulty concentrating; and I can work a full day without getting tired. I almost feel like I'm not sick anymore, I can't wait to test my blood in 3 months! I feel that the Natcell was the key as I received it first and have only used the supplements four of the eight days. After feeling the immediate affect on my thymus gland and assistance in helping my liver regenerate with the Natcell products, I want to also assist my adrenal gland, which I'm sure has been weakened trying to fight this disease during it's incubation period. I have decided to incorporate the Natcell Adrenal into my program, and I ordered it today. About your line of supplements, after reading your book and others, I had went to the vitamin stores and purchased some of the supplements recommended. After I received your package I planned to finish what I had already purchased then start with yours, however after comparing products I literally looked at what I had bought as junk. Your products ingredients, and manufacturing procedures were superior to what I had bought at the health food store, because the supplements target and enhance the immune system and support the liver. They are just what I am looking for. In general, as I said I am stunned. I feel tremendously lucky that I found your web site and very thankful that you took the time to answer my questions. Had I not talked with you when I did, I most likely would be getting ready to start my combo therapy in 2 weeks. When you're sick and they tell you that you have a very serious disease with a very small chance for a cure and you can feel it taking over your body, you'd give anything for your health back. Your program has given me so much hope for the future. Thank you from the bottom of my heart. I'll keep you informed, as my new blood tests will be taken in 3 months.

Sincerely,
Bob

## My Dad's Diabetic Condition Seems to be Improving.

Hi Lloyd,

My Dad's diabetic condition seems to be improving by using the Natcell Pancreas & Thymus. We're still not sure if it the Natcell or not, but my Dad's blood sugar levels have dropped from 230 to 130, which is from fairly high to almost normal. He's only used two bottles of each, but he says overall he feels better. We're testing levels everyday. I am envious of his ability to test his levels so easily; I wish I had a quick test for my AST, ALT, & Viral Load so I could check them everyday. I know it's not your area of expertise, but I'm hoping through your studies and affiliations with many doctors and your clients that you may have some information that could help him with his condition.

When we talked last you mentioned a product similar to the organic glandular thymus. I think it was a pancreas extract. We are interested in it and anything else you might have or know of that could improve his diabetes. I listened to the radio show the other day. It was good to hear you.

Take care,<br>Bob Bartholomew

# EIGHT

## Book Reviews on Amazon.com

The gigantic Internet bookseller Amazon.com carries my book *Triumph Over Hepatitis C*, and has posted numerous favorable reviews of the book on their web site:

### August 22, 2000–Pop Singer YVONNE ELLIMAN Praises Lloyd Wright's *Triumph Over Hep C*

I've seen my dear friend go from standing at death's door to being a vital and healthy man again. He did it by following a program that he has since written into his book, *Triumph Over Hepatitis C.*

Having been in the rock-and-roll business in the crazy 70's, I witnessed a lot of abusive behavior by people I admired. Some of those people are no longer with us but many of them, like Eric Clapton (whose band I was in for four years), turned their lives around and totally cleaned up their acts.

Without the help that's available to people who need it and ask for it, I doubt many of us would have succeeded. For alcoholics and drug addicts there is AA and NA, and various other support groups. For people with hepatitis C, there is good proven advice in Lloyd Wright's book.

If you know anyone who is suffering from this devastating health problem, before you even go near interferon, give them this book. As I have seen in my friend, it WORKS!

Sincerely,
Yvonne Elliman

**June 22, 2001–*Get This Book and Start Your Recovery* by Sharon from Covington, TN**

Reading *Triumph Over Hepatitis C* has given me a whole new outlook on life and a new life. In December 2000, I was diagnosed with hep C. I was fatigued, depressed, confused, and losing my hair.

I went for a checkup and was sent to a liver specialist who said the only successful treatment was interferon. He explained the treatment, the dreadful side effects and the high rate of recurrence of the disease. Not encouraging at all! As I was only experiencing mild symptoms at this point, he suggested I come back to see him in 6 months, unless symptoms worsened. Well, he was the specialist after all, so I decided to wait and see what this silent killer was going to do to my body.

In May 2001, I began researching the web for a cure for my brother's prostate cancer, as I heard there were alternative treatments to surgery. I came across Lloyd Wright's web site "hepatitiscfree.com." Of course, I checked it out. I ordered the book and started taking some of the suggested herbal supplements and modifying my diet.

Within a week, I began noticing a difference in the way I felt. I had follow-up blood work done June 14, 2001. My hep C viral load by PCR dropped 400,000 points, my GGT has dropped 60 points, my ALT dropped 11 points and my iron serum level has dropped 78 points. All this in less than one month of only taking some of the supplements that help your body produce its own natural interferon.

I highly recommend, first, if you have not been tested for hep C to get tested. It is a rapidly growing epidemic.

294

Second, research this disease and read this book. Our so-called liver specialists know little about this silent killer.

As I said, it has changed my life. I am no longer tired all the time, I am sleeping through the night, my thought processes are clearer, and I'm no longer losing my hair. I am looking forward to my next blood test. Get this book and start your recovery today!

### January 15, 2001–*Total Faith–Thank You Lloyd Wright* by Jill from California

It is not often that one is fortunate enough to be helped and guided by someone whose intentions are truly altruistic and from the heart. I feel blessed to have stumbled upon Lloyd Wright's book and now have even more confidence in its healing suggestions after having met the author myself.

Having "procured" the hepatitis C virus from a blood transfusion at age 13, I only discovered that I was carrying this deadly killer in my blood about a year ago at age 32. Not yet sick enough to be tempted to even try the frightening interferon, I felt frozen and powerless in what I could possibly do. I had avoided alcohol since my diagnoses, yet my liver-level enzymes were still increasing way beyond normal.

By chance, someone handed me Lloyd Wright's book and, feeling I should become a bit more familiar with what I now have, I casually began to read his words and soon found myself unable to put it down. In fact, after finishing the book, I immediately phoned Mr. Wright (even though it was 2:30 a.m.!) because I felt certain that from what I had just read that he could very well be my ticket to health through a self-empowering, natural, positive, healing regimen.

Despite his chaotic schedule where he is entirely devoted to helping others 24 hours a day, 7 days a week, Lloyd kindly acquiesced after my insistence to come and see him right away. I found Lloyd Wright to be a beacon of light. He has spent an incredible amount of energy, time, and effort educating himself fully on all aspects and all of the treatments for hepatitis C. Rarely do we meet people such as Lloyd who truly know what they are doing and care enough to help others. He is a guide, an angel, a healer, and a gift to anyone who has hepatitis C.

I have only just begun his program of treatment, but I can already feel a new energy, a positive perspective, and I have total faith in what he prescribes. Additionally, the herbs he recommends are organic, beneficial and life enhancing. Where's the harm? There is none. Only a journey to health.

**February 15, 2000–*Triumph Over Hepatitis C* by Guy Anderson from Redondo Beach, CA**

I was recently diagnosed with hepatitis C and had been feeling afraid and overwhelmed. My wife found Lloyd Wright's book, which I read cover to cover without setting it down. I immediately felt so much better!

The book is a little rough, but very funny, engaging, and full of specific, understandable, useful information. All of the alternative treatments are clearly explained, and they are well supported by historical reference and descriptions of how they work in the human body.

His explanations of what to stay away from and why are equally detailed and enlightening. Try to get the run-of-the-mill doctor in this country to explain ANYTHING as clearly as Mr. Wright has.

I feel hopeful and almost "normal" again. Thank you.

## August 22, 2001–*Triumph Over Hepatitis C: An Alternative Medicine Solution* by Tina from Franklin, TN

I bought this book after finding out that my best friend has hepatitis C. I like the fact that the book is straightforward. Lloyd talks about his ridiculous experiences in dealing with doctors who don't know enough about the disease and certainly don't know how to treat it. He has great, solid ideas on how to improve your health and become hepatitis C–free. It's a tried and true method, it worked for him and he is now free of the disease.

This is a must read for anyone suffering from this debilitating disease and for anyone who needs info in order to help a loved one.

## June 23, 2001–*This Book Saved My Life!* by Katie Glenn from Lexington, S.C.

Hepatitis C is the main reason for a liver transplant. That's what I was told when I was diagnosed in July 2000. I was sent home with a box of needles, Tylenol and another appointment for a liver biopsy. I sat in my car unable to digest the horrible news about my liver. I cried for 30 minutes; I have never been so afraid, ever!

I decided not to do anything until I knew all of the treatments available. After diligent searching, I found a book that I know saved my life; *Triumph over Hepatitis C.*

Lloyd Wright lit the path for the rest of us. His simple approach to getting well was very enlightening to me. I feel as though everyone has a purpose in life, Lloyd Wright knows exactly what we "heppers" are going through, and what we need to survive. It was so obvious to me the minute I started reading the book.

The way Lloyd Wright conveyed the message to the readers; we knew it was for real. He is the most informed human being on the planet when it comes to hepatitis C. I know because my hepatitis C is almost in remission!

I am so thankful for this book, Lloyd. It has changed my life! It gave me hope. My one wish is to someday meet Mr. Wright just to give him a hug for saving my life. I have purchased several of the books and passed them on to others. It is such a light-hearted book to read. Once I started reading I could not put it down, and still have not. I constantly refer to it both as a reference and because it picks me up continuously!

The author of this book takes the reader on a path through his life dealing with this horrific virus, what he did for the virus, blood tests, personal dilemmas and then he so openly shares what would take years for most of us to find out concerning the cleaning and rejuvenation of the liver.

I am pleased to say that I will not need a liver transplant. It is a gift for anyone fortunate enough to have this book placed in the palm of their hands. I mean that with all my heart, and that is what Lloyd Wright did when he wrote this book. He had to; it was his mission in life to follow his heart! I wish I could give this book 10 stars.

Thank you, Mr. Wright

Sincerely, Katie Glenn

### January 25, 2000–*Recovery From Death's Door* by Lyla Duguay, PhD., Malibu, CA

I have known Mr. Wright for a number of years. I observed firsthand his struggle with the ravages of hepatitis C and his frustration with the ignorance and arrogance he experienced with conventional medicine, just like he describes in his book.

I saw how sick he was, and I thought he would die. He describes this in detail in his book. I also saw the effects of the healing process he went through and how he has recovered.

Mr. Wright felt compelled to share his *Triumph Over Hepatitis C* with lay people so they might benefit from what he learned and practiced, without their going through the agony and great financial cost that he experienced.

His book is not a treatise on hepatitis C, but an account that often humorous, of his perilous journey through the conventional approaches to discovering and practicing an alternative and holistic approach with herbs, foods, and other natural supplements.

His book, *Triumph Over Hepatitis C*, is a "no holds barred" authentic account of an ordinary human being in his struggle for survival. Not only does he document the struggle, but he also lists specific remedies.

Throughout the book, the author is able to interject a sense of humor and hope into what would otherwise be just a factual account. I witnessed Mr. Wright going from death's door to becoming well.

I have read his book more than once and recommend it for anyone who has hepatitis. The book is also good reading for anyone who enjoys brutally honest, extremely funny, true-life adventure.

**January 15, 2000–***Alternative Medicine Solution For Hepatitis C* **by Dr. John Finnegan, Malibu, CA**

I reviewed Mr. Wright's book *Triumph Over Hepatitis C* prior to publication and conferred with him on the published edition. I have read the entire volume.

Mr. Wright was a patient of mine beginning in 1996, and I worked with him in developing the remedy he describes in *Triumph Over Hepatitis C*. Mr. Wright describes in his book his condition prior to being diagnosed and presents a copy of his liver biopsy showing chronic hepatitis C as well as significant liver damage from cancer, radiation and chemotherapy.

In accordance with his biopsy results, his liver enzymes were AST panel at 210 (0-41 normal) and ALT panel at 245 (0-45 normal). He was bedridden, and he couldn't tolerate interferon treatment, which he describes in a brutally honest and gut-busting fashion.

He outlines in his book his efforts to adhere to a good nutritional program along with a concentrated effort to take everything in the remedy we developed. He started to feel much better right away, and a year later he was healthy and virus-free. There was no evidence of the virus in his test results. He has been hepatitis C-free for almost three years and his liver-enzymes reading at this time are as follows: AST panel at 23 and ALT panel at 12. Copies of this are included in his book.

Mr. Wright's account of the events he encountered from contraction of hepatitis C to his complete recovery and the remedy that saved his life is a must read for anyone with hepatitis C, cancer, HIV or AIDS. This is a true patient-to-patient testimonial that can save new patients a lot of disappointment, trouble and money. It is a good story that gives real hope for the patient with dire diagnoses. It would not surprise me if this book were made into a movie in record time.

## December 8, 1999–*One Man's Triumph Over Hep C* by WellnessBooks.com

This self-published volume details the experiences of Lloyd Wright, who contracted hepatitis C during a blood transfusion. In the years that followed, the author began what became an almost two-decade-long search for a cure.

Finding the medical community largely unreceptive to alternative treatments, the author embarked on his own research and, using a variety of alternative treatments, is now hepatitis free. The author, no friend of conventional medicine or drug companies, definitely takes sides here and argues for more recognition of alternative remedies for hepatitis.

The last third of the book comprises a list of remedies and their therapeutic effects. Although these alternative remedies may not prove to be a cure-all for everyone, as they were for the author, the author is on the right track in calling for more incorporation and testing of alternative remedies in the conventional medical world. Perhaps this book will help in that effort

Normally books on alternative medicine are boring, although they profess to tell you something that is good for you and your body. This book, however, after the obligatory forewords, begins like a Hunter S. Thompson (*Fear & Loathing In Las Vegas*) tract of frightening dimensions and slowly, slowly levels out into a "Dr. Feelgood" text that anyone who has ever experienced the pain and suffering of hepatitis C can benefit from.

Wright relates how a severe accident, and the blood transfusions thereafter, resulted in his contracting the deadly hepatitis C. His list of the illnesses and maladies to follow, kicking in like falling dominoes, reads like a "Who's Who of Nightmare. "

His accident (read the book for details), which occurred in Malibu in 1979, was the beginning of a trip into the "Black Hole" of incompetent doctors and well-meaning nurses who didn't know themselves what they were looking for that would make him well again. Tested for hepatitis C in July 1991 (the conclusive tests to determine the existence of hepatitis C in a person's body were only achieved in September of 1991!), his results were negative.

Still trying to rid himself of a baffling sickness, in 1994 he made regular weekly visits to a blood bank where his blood was sucked out and supposedly discarded as toxic waste. Murphy's Law kicked in, and this discarded blood mistakenly appeared one day on a shelf with donation blood and was randomly tested. The blood bank sent him a form letter two months (!) later, saying they could no longer accept his blood for donations (!) because he had hepatitis C!

Lloyd Wright has changed his food consumption and lifestyle considerably since 1994. The result has been his survival of an almost-certain death. In his book, he lists the elements (Milk Thistle, Live Cell Therapy, Cat's Claw, Dandelion Root, Aloe Vera, Licorice Root, Alpha Lipoic Acid, Reishi Mushrooms, etc.), which saved his life, and warns against items, which could take your life: Hospitals - the 8th leading cause of Death in America!

Wright's findings are sure to open up some previously closed eyes, ears, and minds.

# *NINE*

# INSIDE PRISON WALLS: GETTING HERBAL THERAPY TO PRISONERS WITH HEP C

Alternative health care touches a broad spectrum of society. I receive numerous letters from prison inmates or their family members requesting copies of my book. Usually, these inmates are given interferon for hepatitis C, or given no treatment at all. Some are allowed milk thistle. At any rate, there is much red tape involved in getting the herbal therapy to the prisoners, if allowed.

Below is a sampling of these letters, which raise the whole issue of the right to engage in alternative therapy when a person is confined to a state penal institution. These sample letters, and my responses, will give the reader a further idea as to the importance of the right to choose one's own therapy. Many of the prisoners I've dealt with are even reading my book so they can plan for their herbal health care once they are released.

## The Right to Engage in Alternative Therapy

Dear Lloyd,

I was told about your successful self-treatment with herbal therapy to cure your chronic hep C infection. I would very much appreciate and welcome any specific information you could send me about this.

Just to give you a brief description of my situation: My name is John and I am currently serving a 25-to-50 year sentence in the N.Y. prison system for first-degree robbery convictions.

I was diagnosed as having hep C in 1993. My condition grew steadily worse. By 1997, I was experiencing greatly elevated liver enzymes (6 to 10 times normal range), and a viral load of 563,000. My liver biopsy test indicated that I had developed grade 2, stage 2 fibrosis.

The prison medical department has refused to give me any treatment at all, so I am in the process of filing a federal lawsuit against them. One issue I would like to raise in my suit is the right to engage in alternative therapy, perhaps herbal therapy, to try and recover from this disease. This is why I need to get the information from you.

I have enclosed a self-addressed stamped envelope with this letter. We are not allowed access to the Internet.

Sincerely,
John

## There is Hope For My Brother When He is Released

Dear Lloyd,

It was a pleasure talking with you today about your book on hepatitis C. Thank you so much for your willingness to send your book to my brother, Greg, at the Ramsey prison in Texas.

Patty spoke so highly of you as a person, as well as your dedication in helping people with this disease. She urged me to call you because of my brother's illness. Thanks again, Lloyd, for your extra efforts in getting your book to Greg. I feel your book would be of interest and value to him since he is considering having the interferon treatment, if and when it is offered to him. Although Greg doesn't have the choice right now to take your treatment, at least he would have the knowledge that other treatment exists, and works. He could choose to stop pushing for the interferon treatment, knowing there is hope for him when he is released.

Sincerely,<br>
Karen

## You Can Just Die in There

Dear Sir,

This is so new to us, but there is a gal that my daughter-in-law in California has become acquainted with whose husband was so ill with hep C that his skin had a kind of transparency. She was worried sick over his condition, but someone who was aware of the situation told her that he should be using milk thistle and that they permit it in prison.

She found out that was true, and he currently is on milk thistle, and is beginning to look and feel a whole lot better.

This gives us hope that our son will be able to use that. Plus, I believe his doctor said that he could use other natural alternatives. Some of the guys he's in with, that have hep C, are not receiving any medical treatment. I guess if you don't have anyone outside that cares and will speak up, you can just die in there. Through his experience and learning, he might be able to help other guys beat this horrible thing!

I just want to say something to you. We think you've got to be a marvelous person to want to help others. Too many people in this day and age are so self-serving and selfish; it's wonderful to know that there are people like you that care.

May God bless you and may you live to be at least 102! Thank you for all your help!

Best regards,<br>
Dolores

## HFI Acts Like Prisoners Deserve This Disease

Dear Mr. Wright,

I would like to purchase your book. I am incarcerated in T.D.C. Texas prison. Diagnosed with B-Core positive. Non-reactive to hep B. Reactive to HCV. My ALT is up and down, a little over normal to a little over 100, 120 or so. I've done a lot of research, and the researchers are all full of bullshit, dude. I wrote HFI, Thelma King about a mastermind plan I have on a bone marrow stem cell culture to handle the hep C epidemic. Here in T.D.C., I could run it down to you because you have the juice. My writing skills are very low, but I am very, very smart. I have A.D.D., but I ain't no dummy.

I've had 2 people read your book and tell me what it's about. Chemistry is a strong area of mine. I understand science oh so very well. Super-charge the bone marrow, main stem cell, and inject the cells in the liver.

I almost died of hep A as a child. I was flat on my back with an IV for 3 ½ months, 24 hours a day. No eating; IV only. So, my theory is, you take a person and give them IV, then total bed rest. No food; total liver at rest. Rejuvenation. Do the injection of bone marrow stem cell, and the only ingestible substance into the body is your balanced juice, your stuff. A person would be living and getting well faster on empty, resting, with new cell growth happening. Can this ever generate an HCV negative?

I'd say it's time for you to get a $50 million grant for research. I get out in 15 months, and I need a cure; plus mankind needs one too. The whole civilization of the human race is dependent on the ability to diagnose and treat problems that arise on a daily basis, with a foresight view. You have that view. Send me your info.

Oh yeah, the interferon. They gave it to a dude here for one year straight. It never worked. It should have been discontinued in six weeks after lab results. But U.T.M.B. overloaded it because they don't know, #1, and they don't care, #2. The hospital did the orthoscopic look. "Oh my god," she said. "Looks like you are an erupting oil well. How are you alive?" "Oops, we killed another one at Ramsey III Hospital."

John Sealy is our main hospital on all the units. We have third-world-country doctors from Africa and Vietnam, who–through their actions and inactions–let people, inmates, die on a regular basis in prison.

I need to buy your book and fine-tune my mind to what's really happening. A friend of mine brought your book over to me and said, "Hey, check it out. He has really done his homework with the herbs and interferon."

I knew the interferon wasn't working, because a woman I know did fine; then she went bad after a year of being healthy. Now she needs a new liver.

HFI acts like prisoners deserve this disease. I'd like to clinch their Hippocratic Oath and get their funding to you. HA!

Take care,<br>Mark

## The Woes of Interferon; The Problem of Getting Herbal Therapy Inside the Walls

Mr. Wright,

I bought your book and I really enjoyed it. I bought it because my son has hep C and I want him to be better. The only thing is my son is in prison, so he can't have a lot of things sent in, and it has to be sent in by the drugstore. So what I'm asking is, are there any of these herbs in pill form and can be sent? Of course I would have to ask permission from the prison first. But out of your list, are there a few I can buy that might help save his liver until he can get home.

They have put him on interferon 3 times a week, and he said that his joints hurt. He is losing weight fast, and his head hurts a lot. When he eats, he feels sick to his stomach. Oh, you know all of this already; you have been there.

But as a mother, I need to feel that I tried to help him what I could and be there for him. I love my son with a love that is unconditional. Please just kinda point me in the right direction. Thank you for your time.

Claudine

Hello Claudine,

Milk thistle is the most important capsule to get for him. I have several clients in prisons, and many of the doctors will prescribe milk thistle. Second, get him MSM. It makes the joint pain go away in just a few days. It is natural sulfur, and there should not be any problem using it. NADH would be great; it relieves many of the side effects of interferon. Interferon interferes with the neuro-transmitters in the brain, and NADH helps correct that. Dandelion root capsules would be good as well. They help remove the toxins, especially when one is taking interferon. These would be the items I would try to get into the prison for him. They have no harmful side effects. They do not make people stoned, so I hope that the warden will allow them. I will be glad to help if I can.

Thank you,
Lloyd

Dear Lloyd,

Thanks for answering my email so fast. Now I'll do what I have to, in order to get permission to send these to him. You just don't know how much it meant to me for you to even answer my mail.

Thank you,
Claudine

Dear Claudine,

I will need to speak with the warden to see if he will let them in. Also, I may need to speak with the prison doctor. It is usually up to the doctor. If he says okay, then it works.

Lloyd

Dear Lloyd,

I will get on this right away, and I'll be seeing my son on Sunday. I visit him every Sunday. Maybe if he calls on Friday evening, I can get this information from him.

I just can't thank you enough for your help, and I know my son will be surprised to hear that you answered my email. He doesn't know yet.

May God bless you for your help. Thank you again.

Claudine

Dear Lloyd,

This is great. I sure hope we can get these items in.

Lloyd

Dear Lloyd,

I just came from seeing my son, and he was not feeling well. He said his body hurt so much; it was like someone had beaten him up from inside of his body. My son has lost 18 to 19 pounds as of now, so I would like to get these things started soon. Thank you again and God bless you.

Claudine

Dear Claudine,

I will start tomorrow morning. Interferon makes people feel very bad, even worse than one can imagine. Also, most people lose weight while using it.

Lloyd

Dear Lloyd,

I went to see my son on Friday, and he asked if we had heard of anything from the warden. I said I hadn't talked to you for a while, and I would get to it as soon as I could. So we were both wondering what happened, if anything.

Thanks,
Claudine

Dear Claudine,

We talked to the warden's secretary yesterday. We left a message requesting permission to provide milk thistle and some other herbs for your son. My goddaughter did this, as she is very successful at getting her way, much better than I. If we do not hear from them, we will call again. Aunika, my goddaughter, said it sounded like there would not be a problem. We will get where we are going, it just takes a little time.

Happy New Year,
Lloyd

## Comment from Lloyd regarding Claudine's case:

After much contact back and forth, alas the prison did not allow the herbs. But prison officials did allow this young man to have a copy of my book. Hopefully, he will be able to proceed with his alternative health care plan once he is released, or sooner if prison doctors decide to allow it.

# TEN

# In closing - Recipe For Recovery

I believe physicians should lead a carefully designed and skillfully executed "therapeutic waltz," if you will. The physician should strive to be the compassionate and skilled doctor-partner who can move the patient gently through the therapeutic process, understanding their partner's basic needs, fears and emotional perspective.

Doctors owe their patients an opinion based on a well-rounded, thorough education. I ask you to give a copy of this book to every doctor you consult with regard to hepatitis C. Email or call me and I will send you a free replacement. Hopefully this will spread the word to some of the non-believing MDs so we can enlist them in the fight against "The Dragon."

I am a person who found an answer–an answer that has proven successful for 96% of the people who had the persistence to follow the program for several months. In attempting to deal with my own diagnosis of hepatitis C, I consulted with the finest naturopaths and nutritionists I could find, and put together a program that I followed for 18 months. I was certified as cured by a hepatitis C research doctor at UCLA on April 10, 1997.

I am not a doctor, I cannot prescribe drugs or give medical advice. However, I can set forth suggestions that will enable you to treat yourself for hepatitis C:

- Start your healing program with a fast using hyssop tea. Hyssop suppresses stomach acid and gives you energy. Simply drink two or more quarts of hyssop tea per day for 3-4 days. At the

315

same time, eliminate red meat and dairy. Then, begin taking:

- Milk Thistle 400 mg 3 times per day
- Lipoic acid 200 mg 3 times per day
- Selenium 400 mcg per day from all sources
- Dandelion root tea, 1 quart per day, afternoon and evening
- Natcell Thymus 1 vial every other day
- Thymus organic glandular 2 caps 3 times per day
- Properly prepared aloe 4 oz. 3 or more times per day
- Reishi mushroom tea or extract 2 cups a day or 500 mg 2 times per day
- Alfalfa 1 gram 2 times per day
- Milk thistle seed tea, several cups per day
- Cat's Claw tea or capsules 500 mg 2 times per day
- Vitamin B complex as directed on bottle
- Vitamin C to tolerance
- Adrenal organic glandular and or Natcell Adrenal, helps liver cell regeneration.
- NADH, 1 per day (protects the liver from damage by alcohol)
- Licorice root tea or capsules as directed. **Do not use if you have high blood pressure.**
- If you develop blood sugar problems, use pancrease organic glandular and or Natcell Pancreas.
- I have had several people resolve the problem doing this. Blood sugar problems and diabetes are often associated with hep C, especially after interferon use.

While you are healing, go easy on your body. For the first 2-4 days, eat only vegetables and fruit, preferably raw, (either along with or after your fast with hyssop tea). Drink fresh-squeezed juices like carrot, beet and green vegetable. **Don't drink alcohol and avoid fats and sugar. Eat only whole, unprocessed food. Find a good health food store in your area and buy your food there**. If you can afford the extra cost, buy organic foods. Also, see if you can find a farmers' market or fruit and vegetable stand and buy your produce fresh. It is especially important to avoid foods made with hydrogenated oil (like potato chips and French fries). Get cold-pressed oil, primarily olive and sesame, at the health food store and do your own cooking. Avoid raw fish and shellfish, and limit your intake of animal protein.

**Eat a well-balanced diet including carbohydrates, proteins, and fats**. Carbohydrates are divided into two groups: simple carbohydrates and complex carbohydrates. Simple carbohydrates are also called simple sugars and include fructose (fruit sugar), table sugar, lactose (milk sugar), and fruit. Complex carbohydrates include fiber and starches and include vegetables, whole grains, peas, and beans. Complex carbohydrates are much better for your health than soft drinks, desserts, candy, and sugar. Chose health! Chose unrefined foods such as fruit, vegetables, peas, beans, and whole-grain products.

Protein is essential for growth and development. It provides your body with energy and it is necessary for making hormones, antibodies, enzymes, and body tissues. Protein is divided into different amino acids and the body needs all of them. Complete proteins are found in chicken, turkey, pork, beef, fresh fish, cheese, eggs, and milk. If possible, buy grain-fed organic meat and eggs and milk from animals that are raised on organic feed without additives. Incomplete protein is found in foods like grains, legumes, and leafy green vegetables. Complete proteins can be made available to the body by combining foods containing different amino acids, thereby getting everything you need. For example, you can combine beans (legumes) with any grain, such as brown rice. Or, you can combine brown rice with beans, nuts, seeds, or wheat. Try eating whole wheat bread with nut butter or add nuts and seeds to salads and vegetable casseroles. Any combination of grains, nuts and seeds, any legumes (such as beans, soy products, peanuts, and peas) and a variety of mixed vegetables will make a satisfying and complete protein. Yogurt is very good for frequent use.

The body needs fats to provide energy and support growth. However, most Americans eat too much of the wrong kinds of fat causing obesity, high blood pressure, heart disease and colon cancer (among other things). There are three major kinds of fats: saturated, polyunsaturated, and monounsaturated.

Saturated fats are found primarily in animal foods such as whole milk, cream, cheese, meat, and some vegetable oils, including coconut oil, palm kernel oil, and vegetable shortening. Saturated fats are usually solid at room temperature. It is best to eat as little as possible of saturated fats.

Polyunsaturated fats are found in corn, soybean, safflower, and sunflower oils. Fish also contains polyunsaturated fatty acids. These types of fat may actually lower your total blood cholesterol levels, however, they are high in calories. These types of fats should be limited to 10 percent of your total calories.

Monounsaturated fatty acids are found in vegetable oils like olive, sesame, and peanut. These are the best oils to use in cooking.

Some specific foods beneficial for people with hepatitis C are: avocados (terrific liver protection), artichokes (patented in the Netherlands for liver disease because they increase liver function), green leafy foods, raw eggs (blended with orange juice and a dash of Pure Synergy), lemons, Lemon rinds (juice, marinade), alfalfa, Buckwheat (great pancakes, muffins, bread etc.), oatmeal, vegetables, steamed, slightly cooked, parsley and parsley flakes (stuffing, potatoes, topping), celery, chocolate (terrific antioxidant), Reishi, Maitake, and Shitake mushrooms, brown rice, stir-fry vegetables, raw organic diary products, (limited) chicken, turkey, pork, and beef, (all available grain-fed organic), fresh fish, properly prepared aloe vera, organic butter. **NO MARGARINE!**, Bee products, such as bee pollen, bee propolis, royal jelly, raw honey, barley grass, cabbage, ginger, beets, dandelion root and/or greens (great in salad), astragalus, hyssop tea, asparagus, and foods that known to be anti-inflammatory, such as such as turmeric, pineapple, and rosemary (used in aromatherapy, marinade, put in stuffing, mashed potatoes ).

Drink lots of good quality clean water, sweat daily, and walk 900 feet after each meal. Basically, don't eat processed foods–foods that have been through a factory and subjected to heat, cold, or chemicals. **Buy a good cookbook at your local health food store (such as *Nourishing Traditions: The Cookbook That Challenges Politically Correct Nutrition and the Diet Dictocrats)* and learn to cook healthy foods. ALSO, watch for Lloyd Wright's new cookbook with healthy recipes for hepatitis C patients coming out soon.**

319

There is a lot more that can be done, but this is the basic program I used to cure myself of hepatitis C. Anyone can do what I did and heal themselves. Tell your doctor you want to enlist his help in pursuing alternative medicine. I mean make him sit down and listen! He owes it to you and all his patients to open his mind and allow himself to be re-educated. Rebel against your doctor, your insurance company, and your HMO if you have to. I urge you to do this with vigor. It is the only way the system will change. Most of all trust your immune system and your own body. Listen and it will tell you what it needs to heal.

Lloyd Wright

## HOW HEALTHY IS OUR HEALTH CARE SYSTEM?

Commentary by Tom Clunie, D.C.

The stories told in *Hepatitis C Free: Alternative Medicine vs. the Drug Industry: THE PEOPLE SPEAK* dramatically illustrate the benefits of nutrition, herbal supplements and vitamins in addressing health challenges. Just as dramatically, the book illustrates the gross shortcomings of conventional medical care. Medical error is now the third leading cause of death in the U.S., but how many million more lives have been lost or ruined by the active suppression of so-called "alternative" health care? How often has "the need to protect the patient" been a ruse to protect the profits of the medical establishment and pharmaceutical companies?

In my own practice as a chiropractor, I used to be angry with medical doctors when I saw how often they led patients down expensive, dangerous, inappropriate health trails. That is, until I saw how they used these dangerous practices and drugs on their own loved ones! Many times, the wives of M.D.s (often with their children) have visited me surreptitiously and told me of their frustration in dealing with their husbands, who see drugs and surgery as the only viable health care options and everything else to be quackery. I quickly realized that if doctors were being so narrow-minded with their loved ones, they REALLY didn't know any better.

I recall one day when I played hooky from my own education at chiropractic college in Southern California. I visited the University of Southern California Medical School to observe what medical students were studying. I slipped into a couple of classes and later listened to medical students chatting in the lunchroom. I really didn't notice anything too different or unusual until I stepped into the bookstore. There I saw stacks of free binders from pharmaceutical companies, all with their logo boldly emblazon on the covers. I saw stacks of free notepads, again with the drug company logo in the lower right hand corner of every page. I realized that no matter what their health orientation might have been before medical school, after being imprinted every day, year after year with logo after logo, these medical students would arrive at the conscious and unconscious conclusion that drugs = health and health = drugs. They become one and the same.

Medical education and practice has been dominated by the pharmaceutical industry since the early years of the last century, and the public well-being has greatly suffered from health care being essentially limited to drugs and surgery. Doctors, too, are victims of this narrow, restricted approach to health. It is a crucial point for them to arrive at the understanding that they have been brainwashed, and not every doctor is there yet.

Wholistic health means looking at the whole person in their whole environment. It means including–but not limited to–drugs and surgery as a part of health care. It means asking what is the best, most practical, most sensible, safest option for the patient at the time, be it an herb, a change in diet, a chiropractic adjustment, a divorce, counseling, an exercise program, and/or drugs or surgery.

The health care system in this country is itself in dire need of healing. The whole system is bogged down and corrupted by vested interests (such as HMOs and drug companies), and governmental rules and regulations that often do more harm than good. There is also dogmatism at all levels and a public that is only dimly aware of what is going on. Lurking ominously in the background is "Codex Alimentarius," an international attempt–using the new so-called "free trade" agreements–to greatly suppress the sale of natural medicines and vitamin supplements.

Some are calling for a national health care system (socialized medicine) as a solution. I believe this would be a mistake. Putting government completely in charge of health care–while government is still controlled by corporate interests–would only make the bad we have now worse. Our ailing health care system is itself a symptom of an ailing political-economic-social system that is in dire straits. I think the best thing we can do at this time is get government out of our health care system as completely as possible. Separation of health care and government! The common law principles of contract/fraud would be far superior in protecting patients. A Health Freedom Act could free patients, doctors, healing organizations, and research groups to pursue the highest health goals without fear from a misdirected, zealous, gun-for-hire government. The cost of health care would drop dramatically as real alternatives become available. Too scary? Too much freedom? With medical error being the third leading cause of death in the United States, what do we have to lose?

So, given the fact that we are living in a health care "dark age," what can you as a health care consumer do to protect yourself and your family?

BE ASSERTIVE!

EDUCATE AND INFORM YOURSELF!

READ THIS BOOK AND PASS IT ON TO OTHERS!

READ THESE BOOKS TOO:

*RACKEETERING IN MEDICINE* by James Carter, and *POLITICS IN HEALING* by Daniel Haley
(These two books outline the medical monopoly's historical assault on "alternative medicine)

*PRESCRIPTION FOR NUTRITIONAL HEALING* by Phyllis A. Balch, CNC and James F. Balch, M.D. (great resource for personal health information and alternative approaches).

There are many approaches to healing and you may have to pursue several before you find the one (or combination) that works for you: chiropractic, nutrition, homeopathic, acupuncture, various body and mind methodologies, as well as conventional allopathic medicine. Don't expect success the first time you try. Be open, persistent, and discerning. Given the current chaos in health care, you have to become your own best health care advocate. Taking responsibility for your own health may not be simple or easy, but you could save your own life or the life of someone you love.

Tom Clunie, D.C.
550 Water St., F4
Santa Cruz, CA 95060

## MESSAGE FROM A SURVIVOR:
### 90% decrease in viral load!

This is to all of you suffering with hepatitis C, especially those of you whose progress in recovery is slow. I was diagnosed with hep C in February of 1999, and considering that I had a friend who had just completed 18 months of pure hell on interferon, I told my doctor that unless he said I would be dead in 5 years without it, I wanted to try to find a better way. Luckily he agreed with me. Referring to interferon he said, "It's nasty stuff."

At this time, my liver enzymes were elevated and my viral load was 62,620,000. I had sold my business of seven years because I was very sick. I started taking some herbs and supplements, and by October of 1999 my viral load was 39,610,000, and I was feeling a bit better. So I slacked off on the herbs. By February of 2000, I was back up to 66,710,000, and I felt like I was dying. So once again, I began taking more herbs.

By September, I had found Lloyd Wright's web site on the Internet, and I had finally gotten it through my thick skull that there really was something to the herbs. I began taking as many of Lloyd's products as I could, and I noticed a dramatic increase in my energy level. Also, my liver stopped aching, my skin stopped itching, and in time, virtually all of my symptoms either went away or diminished tremendously.

I have really struggled from time to time with taking everything like I'm supposed to and with wanting to just give up and die. (I'm only 47 years old.) It's a struggle to discontinue my bad habits and eat healthier. All along the way, Lloyd has encouraged me to keep at it and remember that I had an extremely high viral load and was very sick, so it might take longer for me to recover. I had my blood tested the other day and my liver enzymes are fine. Best of all, my viral load is (are you ready for this?) 6,287,740, which is about a 90% decrease! I am thrilled and so encouraged. I want to get rid of this virus, and I believe I will. It's all up to me. I am the only one who can get up in the morning, go to the freezer, and take out that little brown vial. I am the only one who can make those time-consuming, all-important teas and swallow all those pills all day long. I decided in the very beginning to take matters into my own hands, but sometimes it's very difficult to have the discipline to keep at it. One time I complained to my Doctor about how hard it was to take all this stuff, and he reminded me of the alternatives. He is as supportive as an MD can be. He also told me that he'd love to have something else to offer his hep C patients (besides combo therapy) and that he'll be real interested to see what happens with me.

When he gave me the results of my viral titer the other day, he told me that it will not be medically significant until it's under 2,000,000. "That's when people respond more favorably to interferon," he said. But that is not why I am doing this, and a 90% decrease is VERY significant to me.

I hope my progress will inspire others to keep at it, be patient, and give it time. I look at this much the same way as I do fertilizers. If you use chemical products, you will get pretty fast results–a green lawn in 2 days–but it doesn't last. It's only cosmetic, and you have to keep doing it over and over. If you use organic products, it will take longer to get the desired result, but you will end up not only with a healthier, greener lawn, you'll also have a healthy root system, without putting deadly chemicals into the environment. It's not a quick fix; it's a process that takes time and patience. I do believe now that all good things come to those who wait.

Sincerely,<br>
Jane

# TRIUMPH OVER HEPATITIS C

# A NON-PROFIT ORGANIZATION

For information regarding tax deductible contributions or product sales and ordering, contact Lloyd Wright:

Email: Lloyd@hepatitiscfree.com
Web site: www.hepatitiscfree.com
**Toll Free 866 hepcfree • (866) 437 2373**

As a courtesy to my readers, I am happy to provide everything necessary to follow my program at wholesale prices. This is done for your convenience. I had a very difficult time finding the best quality items when I was sick, and I was charged outrageous prices.

Please send your tax-free donation to:

Lloyd Wright
P.O. Box 6347
Malibu, Ca. 90264

Make your donation checks payable to "Triumph Over Hepatitis C." EIN # 95-4820285

Thank you for your support!